FREE TO DANCE

TRACEY JERALD

Just Dance!

xoxo,
Tracey Jerald

Sigrid ♡

Just Daniel!
xoxo,
Amanda
Smith

FREE TO DANCE

To Sue.
Since you were the first to tell me you fell in love with the Freemans, I
thought it was appropriate the first book of the next generation belongs
to you.
I love you more.

ALSO BY TRACEY JERALD

Midas Series

Perfect Proposal

Perfect Assumption

Perfect Composition (Summer 2021)

Perfect Order (Fall 2021)

Amaryllis Series

Free - An amaryllis Prequel

(Newsletter Subscribers only)

Free to Dream

Free to Run

Free to Rejoice

Free to Breathe

Free to Believe

Free to Live

Free to Dance

Free to wish:

An 1,001 Dark Nights Short Story Anthology Winner (Re-Issue with additional content - Summer 2021)

Glacier Adventure Series

Return by Air

Return by Land

Return by Sea

Sandalones

Close Match

Ripple Effect (Available on all platforms)

Lady Boss Press Releases

Challenged by You

Unconditionally with Me (Summer 2021)

PLAYLIST

Lady Gaga: "Just Dance"
Katy Perry: "Firework"
Lady Gaga: "Born This Way"
Demi Lovato: "Sorry Not Sorry"
Maroon 5, Christina Aguilera: "Moves Like Jagger"
P!nk, Chris Stapleton: "Love Me Anyway"
Niall Horan: "Slow Hands"
Imagine Dragons: "Bad Liar"
The Chainsmokers, Coldplay: "Something Just Like This"
Sia: The Greatest
Rihanna, Mikky Ekko: "Stay"

THE LEGEND OF AMARYLLIS

There are variations regarding the legend of how amaryllis flowers came to be. Generally, the tale is told like this:

Amaryllis, a shy nymph, fell deeply in love with Alteo, a shepherd with great strength and beauty, but her love was not returned. He was too obsessed with his gardens to pay much attention to her.

Amaryllis hoped to win Alteo over by giving him the one thing he wanted most, a flower so unique it had never existed in the world before. She sought advice from the oracle Delphi and carefully followed his instructions. She dressed in white, and for thirty nights, appeared on Alteo's doorstep, piercing her heart with a golden arrow.

When Alteo finally opened his eyes to what was before him, he saw only a striking crimson flower that sprung from the blood of Amaryllis's heart.

It's not surprising the amaryllis has come to be the symbol of pride, determination, and radiant beauty. What's also not surprising is somehow, someway, we all bleed a little bit while we're falling in love.

PROLOGUE
MARCO

I'm holding a piece of card stock in my hand that closes the final door on a very cherished part of my past. A part I'm not entirely certain I'm ready to let go of.

You are cordially invited to join the celebration of two hearts uniting in marriage...

Placing the card down, I stand up and move to the bank of windows that overlook the dance floor of Redemption. My redemption, I remind myself. So far from the long-ago rooms in Paris where...

I whirl around and pick up the invitation again.

...Corinna Freeman and Colby Hunt.

"*Ma chère amie*, I could not be happier for you," I say aloud. "Your Colby chased all those demons from your eyes."

"He did, didn't he?" Somehow, I'm not surprised when I hear her voice. "Now what do we have to do to chase the ones from yours, Marco?" Corinna's arm slides around my waist naturally. Just because we were once lovers doesn't mean we're not friends. And surprisingly, it's a strong friendship her fiancé cultivated through the months of hell she survived.

Now, I not only count my blessings I didn't lose her when I realized she could never let him go from her heart, but I now count him among the few people I call friends.

"Does your fiancé know you are here with me? I have witnessed the fists he has thrown on your behalf, Cori," I tease.

She makes a scoffing sound. "Right now, he's recommending security upgrades—for a nominal fee, of course—to Louie. You should be very scared, Marco. This may cut into your profits significantly if we leave the two of them alone for too long. I believe they're starting to develop a bromance."

Her words cause me to toss my head back and roar with laughter. Once I have myself under control, I ask her a question I've been dying to know all these long years. "How did you know I had demons?"

"I didn't. Then."

My jaw falls open. "And yet you trusted me enough to..."

Corinna steps in front of me. There's enough of the woman I believed I was falling in love with still there for me to remember days long past. But she's changed, and I don't just mean the cut of her hair or her eyes—which shine gold almost constantly with happiness.

More than the wedding invitation on my desk, the glow surrounding Corinna reiterates the fact she's no longer mine. She's grown from the lost young lady I crashed into one day on a city street into the confident woman before me. Her soul isn't lost any longer. She no longer needs redemption.

But I do. I always will.

Reaching out, I tweak her chin. "It matters not. I'm honored to be your friend, Corinna."

Anxiously, she asks, "And you'll come to the wedding?" She reaches for my hand. "Marco, you were—are—one of my closest friends. The day won't be the same without you there."

"Are you sure you want me there with senators and the other sort of people who will be on your guest list?" I probe. "Ah, I don't need to ask you to speak. Your eyes are very expressive, *chérie*. They turn such an ugly brown at my words."

"We try to avoid that, Marco. Unfortunately, Cassidy taught her to throw food to relieve her anger," a deep male voice comes from the door.

With a smile, I let Corinna stew and hold out my hand to shake Colby's. *"Mon pote, bonjour." I greet Colby as a friend, because through Corinna, that's what he's become.*

"I'd say it was good to see you too except that crap that spewed from your mouth," Colby reprimands me.

I wander over to the window near Corinna. "It's acceptable for so many people to mingle here in the dark. In the light?"

"Then they decide to not come. This is my wedding, Marco. And if they don't like my guest list, they're not welcome. I only care if family comes anyway," Corinna says forcefully.

I turn slightly and witness Colby dropping a kiss on top of Corinna's head. I feel a pang in the region of my chest where my heart is— not because it's Corinna, but because I wonder what it would be like to be loved that unconditionally, where there's no judgment for the past and without reserve.

"Come to the wedding, Marco. You never know how one yes can change your life," Corinna cajoles.

With a sigh, I turn to pick up the RSVP card to accept, when I catch sight of a picture of Corinna and me intermixed on the credenza of photos. She's right, I muse as I accept the invitation to their wedding. It's amazing how saying yes to one thing can change your life.

Even if it's a dance.

After all, haven't I spent years observing that here at Redemption?

1

MARCO
SEVEN YEARS LATER

Redemption. So many rush here to seek it. Whether it's with a stiff drink or through the pulsating beat on the dance floor, I find myself amused every night by the people who think redemption is something they can buy with an ostentatious cover charge.

Of course, I'm not foolish. I perpetuate the illusion that anything can be bought at Redemption for a price whether it's sex or your soul. Wandering around the upper floor of the club I've owned and operated for a dozen years, I nod at a few celebrities I recognize in the VIP section when my phone vibrates in my pocket. Slipping it out, my lips curve into a rare smile when I glimpse the name associated with the text on the screen. It's a smile I reserve for only three women in my life: my two sisters-in-law and a woman I once thought I could find my own personal ever after with.

Corinna Freeman.

No. Mentally, I correct myself. Corinna Freeman-Hunt. Now blissfully married, Corinna, her husband Colby, and their assorted family members have enjoyed spending time at Redemption on many occasions. But what I've found peculiar is that even after knowing what his wife once meant to me, Colby still welcomed me into the Freeman fold after an excruciating time long in Corinna's past.

Quickly typing in my password, I expect her text to be nothing more than the usual edict to haul my ass to the suburbs to make an appearance at a "Freeman Family Dinner." Vaguely amused, I recall the time I told my sister-in-law, Broadway star Evangeline Brogan, she needed to pitch the idea about have a musical written about these events. But as I read Cori's text, my jaw drops, and all thoughts of Corinna's brother's ridiculous antics fly right out of my mind.

Jenna is getting married!!!

My response is swift. *And those heathens you call brothers-in-law didn't murder him? I'm impressed.*

A bunch of laughing emojis come back before she replies, *I think Jake was in too much shock.*

Why do I detect a story there?

Because you know us too well?

I grip the edges of my phone. There was a time when I thought knew Corinna better than anybody did, including her siblings. I cared for her deeply, though my heart never quite took the kind of fall over the edge that it never recovered. Our relationship evolved into exactly what it was supposed to be.

Friends.

But there are moments like this where I miss the closeness of intimacy between us, hell, between myself and any woman. It's not that I haven't had lovers since Cori; it's that none of them have touched that part of me I barricade.

Coming out of my stupor, my fingers fly across the keyboard. *Ma chère amie, any man who claims to understand that family is a liar. We merely pretend to protect ourselves from ongoing suffering.*

Again, I get back a bunch of laughter. And I smile again. Then, the expected *Want to come next Saturday for dinner at the farm before we move the insanity to Nantucket for the actual event?*

That quickly? I'm honestly shocked.

According to Jenna, they've spent too many years apart. I know the feel-

ing. The dreamy-eyed emoji she sends to accompany this text would hurt if I still had feelings for Corinna, but all it does is make me shake my head over how desperately in love she is.

With the right man.

But I regretfully have to decline a night of amusing myself amid the insanity of the Freeman family. *I can't. Simon and E's new show is opening that night on Broadway. Bristol and I will be sitting front and center.*

Well tell them to break a leg! Talk soon!

Absolument.

Wow. I slip my phone back in my pocket as I continue my circle around the sky bridge past one of the dancers clad in a skimpy bit of nothing that reflects the lights bouncing off the strategically placed chandelier nearby. She offers me a come-hither smile I turn down with nothing more than a dip of my lips downward. I learned early on in this business never to mix my personal proclivities with my employees. It made for some ugly scenes in my early years I care not to repeat.

Moving over to my number two, Louie Scott, who is lounging in the doorway guarding the exclusive VIP entrance like he does every night, I note briefly the well-dressed people eager to get in. Some begin screaming my name to get my attention, but I singularly ignore the antics. Instead, I murmur, "Did you hear the news?"

Louie grins. "You met a woman and fell in love?"

I roll my eyes because it's a long-standing joke between us. After coming so close with Cori, I haven't found a woman I cared enough about to peruse with that single-minded intent. "You wish."

"I do. Maybe you'd be happy again." Seriousness coming from the burly man temporarily stuns me.

"Well, someone found love."

"Not you," he clarifies.

"Louie, if I did, don't you think you'd be one of the first people to know?" My voice is laced with exasperation. In the last ten years, other than my brother, Louie's been my closest friend. Along with

Cori. Speaking of whom— "Little Jenna Madison's getting married. She must be what? Twenty-one?"

Louie belts out a laugh so hard, it echoes off the dark cavernous entrance. "Twenty-one? Try twenty-five, Marco."

I scrub my hand over my head. "Christ, I'm getting old."

Louie grins and the flash of gold attached to his front tooth winks at me. "Seasoned. Just like a fine wine or a beautiful woman, you just keep getting better with age."

"You're like six months younger than me," I protest.

"I'll always be six months younger than you. Which means when you hit the big 4-0 next year, I'll have six uninterrupted months of cracking old jokes at your expense."

"Tell me again why I keep you around?"

"Because like your family, I want nothing from you other than your sparkling personality," Louie immediately replies.

And it's true. It's also one of the main reasons I've missed having a woman like Corinna in my life. We met when we collided into each other—literally—after she was coming out of Zabar's on Broadway holding bags of groceries. I wasn't paying attention and slammed right into her. But the minute her golden eyes met mine, I knew I'd found a treasure. I just was meant to protect it, not to keep it.

Pulling myself from a past that can't be changed, I wonder aloud, "What do you think about offering up Redemption to Jenna for her bachelorette party?"

Louie gapes at me. Staggering to his feet, he grips my shoulders in his hands. Topping my six-foot height by an easy six inches, he has to lean down to meet my eyes. "Eyes appear to be dilating correctly."

"You're an ass," I tell him succinctly.

"And you've obviously lost your mind," he retorts. "You've been there, Marco. They're not just stories or fantastical lore. If we set that family loose on Redemption during Jenna's party, this club will never be the same."

A wicked smile crosses my face. "Well, we did say we were looking to spice things up a bit," I remind him of a conversation we had during our last business meeting.

"Not by allowing the customers to dance on the tables!"

I cede the point. "So, there will have to be some ground rules."

"In writing, or I'll pull out zip ties to strap their sweet asses to the booth."

I grin. "Let me find out the family's plans from Cori before you start ordering supplies to restrain the sisters."

"It's not the sisters I'm worried about. It's their damn brother who is the epicenter of all the trouble in that group!" Louie's hand flaps up and down like his aging grandmother.

I open my mouth to make the comparison but hold myself back. I don't need him pulling some prank on our clients like demanding they wear bracelets to determine what sex they're going to hit on once they get inside Redemption—a trick he pulled off on Corinna's husband during their courtship. Turning on my heel, I flick my wrist out and head back into the inky portal leading toward the crushed velvet drapes that hide the inner sanctum of Redemption to the outside view.

"Hey, Marco?" Louie calls.

Pausing, I turn.

"You know I'm just giving you a hard time, man. I love Cori and her family. Whatever you need. Even if it means hiring personal security for the night." The last he adds as a personal aside.

"I'm pretty certain we can get a discount on that," I remind him wryly as Cori's husband and brothers-in-law own one of the most prestigious investigations and security firms in the nation.

Louie's face brightens. "I forgot all about that. Then yeah, let's do this. Security needs an overhaul anyway. Maybe Keene will consider giving us a discount."

Chuckling, I duck behind the velvet and go back to what I know how to do best—hiding inside the world I created so I don't have to feel anything more than what I choose to brush up against my skin: the frantic pulse of the music, the almost tangible pursuit between the men and the women as they seek out companionship for a night or more. And above all, the bodies of the hundreds of people on the dance floor as they cut loose and just dance.

What else do I need beyond this? I ask myself as I make my way down to the dance floor. Arching a brow, I take the hand of a familiar partner and try to forget about the pain near the region near my heart when I realize this is all I have even as time passes on.

2

LYNNE

There's something to be said for flying first class, I think as the handsome steward passes me a glass of complimentary whiskey. Taking a small sip, I study the email on my screen before forwarding the message to my boss from 34,000 feet in the air as I cross the Atlantic.

Client agrees with my recommendation. Sell.

Her thumbs-up reply is immediate. And I smile thinking of the delicious commission we're going to earn off that trade. Maybe I'll treat myself to a new handbag to go with the dress Jenna's stepmother, Emily, is making for me for the bachelorette party in a few days.

Another Emily Freeman original to add to my collection. My lips curve when I recall the summer Em and Jenna's dad, Jake, fell in love. Not only did I gain a lifelong best friend in Jenna when we both worked for the only decent coffee shop on Nantucket Island, I managed to gain a family who loves me for exactly who I was then: insecure, overwhelmed, and overweight.

But one afternoon with Em and her sister Corinna changed my perspective about myself and my body for the better. No, I correct myself, for the best.

Smoothing my hand down the leg of my tailored pants, I won't claim I've turned into some nutrition guru, and I haven't met a caramel macchiato I can resist yet, but I realized I'm beautiful. I have curves I now celebrate instead of hiding, but the best one resides between my ears.

After suffering years of emotional pain at the hands of my parents by not doing my best to become their walking, talking image of a Bradbury, I turned my back on my familial ties. I eschewed the Ivy League education they dangled over my head and went to UConn with Jenna on a full ride.

Funny how a perfect GPA and GMAT scores plus a raving recommendation from my boss—Ryan Lockwood, a shipping billionaire who happens to have one of the kindest souls I've ever known—helped open the door to a dream. Since I interned all four years for Ryan at Lockwood Industries, I felt no shame crying as he danced me around his Manhattan office the day I received my acceptance letter to the renowned London Business School. Then again, I think that might have something to do with the amount of champagne we drank after I called and told my parents I was moving to London.

It was Ryan who sent Jenna over for my birthday that fall. And his husband, Jared, who happened to be in London in time to pick me up for Christmas that first year.

And when I was finishing my capstone, Ryan declared I needed practical experience. With a smile, I check the balance of the scholarship account I still manage to this day. From the first million he gave me to invest, it's grown to over a hundred million dollars in just under four years. But I'll never forget his words as I stammered out my gratitude. "For fun, Lynne. I consider it critical you get some practical experience. Much better than those textbooks you're burying your nose in."

Now, the money funds scholarships at dozens of universities. It's been my job the last few years to read the applications, determine the expenditures, and allocate the funds.

But I felt something driving me to make a change.

Perhaps it was meeting the woman recently dubbed the "Queen

of Wall Street," Bristol Brogan, at an FWA meeting in New York, but I began to want more from my career.

Talking about it with Ryan turned out to be easier expected.

"Well, of course, Lynne! What the hell do you think you went to school for? To review proposals for me the rest of your life?" Ryan tossed a file on the glass-topped conference table with a flick of his wrist. His handsome face contorted. "Please tell me you haven't been holding yourself back because of some convoluted obligation to Lockwood."

I fiddled with the pen in front of me. "I wouldn't say that exactly."

He let out a sigh as he dropped into the chair next to me. "What would you call it?"

"Fear that I would lose all of you," In my head I knew I'd never find acceptance like I had with the Freemans and their spouses.

Ryan roared with laughter before reaching over and laying his hand on top of mine. "Trust me, even if the rest of us didn't love you the way we do, Phil never lets someone he adopts into our little clan go." Ryan mentioned the name of his most outrageous brother-in-law.

A smile started to grow because it was no less than the truth. "God, that's a perfect way to describe him. Phillip Freeman-Ross, clan chief."

"Never tell him that, or I'll refuse to give you a reference. Now, Lynne, tell Bristol you're taking that job. It's what you worked for."

That was six months ago. And between wrapping up my work for Lockwood Industries and learning my responsibilities for Brogan Limited—Bristol Brogan's boutique investment firm that's kicking the boys' club of Wall Street back into their locker rooms—I've barely spent any time in New York.

I've traveled the Orient to Dubai, from LA back to New York. Luckily, a few of my trips have intersected with Jenna's or I'd be flipping out about her and Professor O'Roarke. Damnit, I mentally curse myself—Finn. I just hope I don't screw up during the maid-of-honor speech and call him that.

Then again, I doubt either Jenna or Finn would care. They're too busy making up for "bloody ridiculous lost time. And all due to my black pride, Lynne," Finn admitted to me in a bar in Dublin.

As the pilot announces our descent into JFK, I put away my laptop and wonder briefly about how the next few weeks are going to play out. Fortunately, I'm not expected in the office in the next week unless it's a dire emergency and then not after that until after the wedding is over.

But first things first. Get off this plane, get my stuff, and head to Connecticut.

"I'M SO excited you're here!" Jenna's arms squeeze the breath out of me the minute I alight from my Jag at the Freeman farm in Collyer, Connecticut, later that night.

Laughing, I return the embrace just as fiercely. "Like I'd miss a second of this."

"Finn and I were worried your plane would be delayed," she explains as we walk up to the doors beyond which I know chaos is going to reign.

Stopping short, I admit, "It's still hard not to let Professor O'Hell Yes slip out."

Jenna tosses her long blonde hair back. "Oh, Lynne, please do," she begs. "Especially in front of the family."

Then the lilting voice of the man himself intrudes, causing me to flush hotly. "You just want to role-play naughty schoolgirl again, Jenna," Finn accuses before he bends down to brush his lips across my cheek. "It's good to see you, Lynne."

"You too, Prof—"

He raises a brow.

"Finn," I correct myself. Glaring at both of them, I state, "Why is it I have no problem talking to wealthy people all over the world, but hanging with the two of you for a few minutes makes me feel all tongue-tied?"

Jenna opens her mouth, but Finn shuts it effectively by pressing his lips on hers. "Perhaps because here you're you? Out there"—he waves his hand in the direction of my car—"you perfected who Lynne Bradbury should be. There's no need to maintain that armor with family. Especially with a group of people who were discussing dancing on the furniture. Will they really do that?"

"Yes!" Jenna and I answer simultaneously before we burst into laughter.

"I know I've said it before, but welcome to the family, Finn," I laugh.

"I think I'll go find safety with the men," he jokes. He squeezes Jenna's shoulder, nods at me, and makes his way back the way he came.

"Good luck with that!" Jenna yells after her fiancé.

He turns and gives her a wolfish smile that immediately transports me back to his class five years ago at UConn.

"Damn, the man still has it," I mutter the minute the heavy door shuts.

"Tell me about it." Jenna's voice is dreamy.

I shove her. "Lucky bitch."

She laughs, hooking her arm through mine and leading me up to the porch. "What? No one currently keeping you warm at night?"

"When would I have time? I'm too busy traveling."

"That didn't stop me. And look where I ended up," Jenna reminds me just before she opens the door to a cacophony of sound that might terrify an outsider. But for me, it's just the sounds of home.

A family born of the will to survive, Phil, Cassidy, Emily, Alison, Corinna, and Holly Freeman moved to Connecticut with the intent of escaping the past that seemed to haunt them in the South. None of them expected to find their perfect match in their husbands, or the additional family members who have been welcomed with an open heart.

I feel strong arms wrap tightly around my legs when we enter the great room, and scooping up the little girl with corkscrew ringlets, I place a smacking kiss on Jenna's adopted-sister's cheek. "Who's going to look beautiful in her flower girl dress?"

Talia shrieks, "Me!" But then her full lips pout.

Shifting her to my hip, I stroke her satiny cheek. "What is it, Princess?"

Grabbing my face, she peers into my eyes intensely. "I should go to the cackle-ette party."

Confused, I swivel us both to Jenna, who plucks her sister away with ease. "Bachelorette," Jenna corrects. "And no. It's for adults."

Talia flings her arms out wide, almost taking out Keene and Ali's oldest daughter, Kalie, in the process. Kalie shrugs as if it happens all the time, which it likely does, before dashing down the hall yelling, "Come out, come out, wherever you are!"

Talia's pout almost reaches her chin. I tug on the lower lip lightly before I reason, "If you stop giving Jenna a hard time about the party, I promise to take you swimming when we get to the island."

Talia's hand dramatically moves to her forehead. "I s'pose."

Behind her, my best friend stifles a giggle at her baby sister's antics. "Come on, Trouble. Let's go find Mama."

"How about we go find Aunt Cori first?" Talia wheedles.

Spotting Em across the room in the kitchen with her sisters, I bop Talia on the nose. "Fortunately for you, they're both in the kitchen."

We make our way through Jenna's enormous family toward the kitchen, getting stopped every few feet when each of Jenna's uncles welcomes me "home." I'm basking under the warm reception until Talia reaches over as I'm being embraced by Phil and shakes my shoulder. "Hurry, Lynne. Please?"

Phil's shoulders shake. "I find it to be poetic justice that Em's daughter is a complete chatterbox."

"She's desperately trying to get to Cori," I explain.

"But just for snuggles," Jenna manages with a straight face

"Ah. Well, we can't have that." Phil resolutely plucks Talia out of Jenna's arms and drives ahead into the kitchen. "Make way! Child in desperate need of sweets!"

"Talia doesn't need..." Em begins to protest.

"I wasn't talking about her," Phil deadpans.

"Oh, so you're finally owning your emotions. That's a big step, brother," Ali snarks.

"You know the rules, Phil," Cassidy chides.

"If someone starts dessert early, none of the kids will eat," Corinna mutters as she spreads frosting around a cake. Her hand rests on her protruding stomach.

Phil asks, "Should you still be doing that in your condition?"

"Better me at seven months pregnant than you any day of the week," Corinna retorts.

Stepping aside, he jerks his head at me and Jenna. "Well, what about letting Jenna and Lynne help? I mean, if they're old enough to get married and travel the world, they're old enough to..." His words are drowned out by the excited shrieks led by Emily.

"Lynne! You made it!" Em's blonde curls dance as she wraps me in an enormous hug that I felt for the first time ten years ago on the sandy beach in Nantucket. Back then, I was overwhelmed and intimidated. Now, I'm so much more because of the way they opened their hearts.

Starting with Jenna.

"I just got here. Like I told Jenna, there was no way I was missing a second of this."

"Where are you staying?" Ali demands.

"Jenna said here," I begin, and that sets off an argument over which sibling I'll be crashing with until we head to Nantucket next week to the beach house of supermodel Danielle Madison and Brendan Blake to get ready for Jenna and Finn's ceremony—the same place Em and Jenna's father got married.

I feel a kiss pressed to the side of my head before Cassidy whispers, "Welcome home."

And before I can say a word in return, someone puts Brendan's latest hit on the stereo. Ali whoops and yells, "I call dibs on the end table!" sprinting across the room.

Holly brushes her cheek against mine, reaching for her camera.

Cassidy and Em both pat Corinna's arms consolingly as they leap onto the long farm table. Corinna slinks to the corner with a sigh while Phil holds on to Talia.

Jenna and I exchange quick glances before we boost ourselves up onto the bar.

We're all belting out the lyrics to a song about grabbing hold of your family tight—a song we'll likely hear live in just under two weeks—when the back door opens and Finn yells, "Bloody fecking hell, the stories are true!"

Jake clasps Finn's shoulder and confirms, "Last chance to bail, Finn."

Jenna reaches down for a plastic cup and, in time to the song, pelts her father in the head.

No, it's not good to be home; it's great.

3

LYNNE

"Wait." I hold up my arm which is imprisoned by straight pins. "I thought we were doing the bachelorette party at Tide Pool?" I name the honky-tonk on the edge of Collyer that has seen more than its fair share of Freeman events over the years, some of which I'm certain will come back and be used as blackmail material later in life.

"That was the plan," Jenna agrees, smoothing her hands over the incandescent blue palazzo pants Em designed for her. Tiny little beads catch the overhead spotlight, sending sparkles of colors across the room. "I love these, Em."

"Thanks. Don't ruin them. They're only basted," she warns.

"Think they'll work at Redemption?" Jenna asks, like the change of plans is a done deal.

"Presumptuous much?" I drawl as Em adjusts the hemline... higher? "Am I going to be able to be able to wear panties with this dress, Em?"

Her sparkling blue eyes meet mine from behind her signature red glasses. Over the years the style has changed, but the color has remained the same. "Absolutely not."

I choke before gasping, "Then how about slipping a girl a few inches if we're striking a pose at the hottest club in the Manhattan area?"

A chuckle from the doorway captures all our attention. Corinna's rubbing her stomach. "Oh, Lynne. If Phil ever heard you say that, you'd never live it down. You'd better be grateful he's out delivering an order."

Realizing what I just said, I groan. "For God's sake, don't tell him!"

"Then let Em do her job." Corinna pushes off the jamb and crosses the room. "She's always known what looks beautiful on you."

I open my mouth but close it on a snap at the firm look in Corinna's golden eyes. "I guess wearing this, I'm not sixteen anymore, am I?" I joke.

Her lips curve. "Hardly that. But at Redemption you'll see people barely wearing things that classify as clothes."

"Klassy with a *K*," Em mutters around a mouthful of pins as she realigns the beaded hem.

Corinna doesn't miss a beat. "And you're going to recognize people who are celebrities in T-shirts and jeans. That's just the way it is."

"Remember how we used to talk about it when these guys or Dani and Brendan would go? Don't you want to see what's inside? Just one time?" Jenna looks so hopeful, I can't refuse her.

With a sigh, I relent. "Where are we all staying in the city that night? Because there's no way we're driving back to Collyer."

Jenna begins to dance on her little platform. I can't help but laugh at her until a telltale ripping sound renders through the room. "Whoops." Her hand reaches behind her just as Phil strolls into the room unannounced.

"Geez, Jenna. Do you have ants in your pants about the wedding? What the hell did you do?"

Before she says a word, I jump in. "She's just excited because she talked me into changing the bachelorette party plans so we can go to Redemption."

Phil turns to Corinna slowly. He gives her the once-over, his eyes lingering on her stomach. Then he starts howling with laughter. "Well, this should be a night to remember."

Em pulls the last pin from her mouth. "That's what I was thinking. Good thing we get everything on film."

Jenna and I exchange confused looks, but before we can ask, Em announces, "Lynne, you're all set. Go ahead and change into your maid-of-honor dress."

Carefully, I step down from the platform to make my way back to the dressing room. As I turn my back, Phil lets out a low wolf whistle. "You look amazing, Lynne. Tell me that number is for the bachelorette party."

"It is," I confirm.

Phil shakes his head before announcing, "Forget being redeemed. We're going to hell."

Em sighs in exasperation. "Well, like we didn't know you were leading the charge there, Phillip. Please."

After a moment, all of us start laughing.

AFTER CAUSING everyone at Amaryllis Events to laugh hysterically when I advised them the owner of Tide Pool was openly relieved we were going to host the party somewhere else, I worked alongside Ali to firm up the logistics. "Here's my thought." I lean forward with my iPad in hand. Cassidy's already given me access to the family calendar so I can coordinate schedules. "If you don't mind your immediate family invading yours and Keene's place in the city—"

Ali interrupts, "Trust me, we're used to that."

I laugh. "Then me and Jenna and our special guest can crash at mine. Our condos are only a few blocks apart in Tribeca."

"I like where you're going with this so far." Ali leans forward and taps her finger against the screen. "Why Thursday?"

"Girls' weekend," I announce.

Ali's lips curve into a sphinxlike smile. "Do we get to dump Phil?"

"If you can manage it."

"I can have someone remove him from the family calendar." Ali's thoughtful. "Damnit, I can't do that to him. He hasn't irritated me in a long while."

I gape at her. "How is that possible?"

Her shoulders rise and fall helplessly. "After you electronically emasculate a man, they're weak. You have to be gentle with them. Unless..." Her nose scrunches like it's sniffing something. "Oh no, he did not." Like a bolt of lightning, Ali shoots for the door and is in the hallway before I can confirm my plans to spend Thursday afternoon at the spa being pampered before we go to the club that night.

Ali lets out an ear-piercing scream. "You didn't! How could you?"

"I thought you were in a meeting." Phil sounds guilty.

"None of us are ever in a meeting that can't be interrupted for Genoa!" Holly yells. Uh-oh. When Holly yells, things are about to go bad fast. I wonder if I can sneak out.

Slipping my iPad into my purse, I'm about to go down the stairs when the conference room door flies open and an infuriated Cassidy and Em storm out. Quickly I head for the front stairs, but then I take refuge back in Ali's office. Corinna's coming up the stairs holding a chef's knife and a tomato with a vicious look on her face.

"You dare?" Corinna breathes.

"Oh, shit." I briefly wonder if I should call Jenna to find out how to handle the situation when Corinna starts scoring the tomato with the edge of the chef's knife.

"I am pregnant with a miniature human. She's obviously Colby's because every night, she plays war games in my stomach. Do you have any idea what that feels like, Phillip?" Corinna shouts as she approaches him. Her fingers clench around the tomato. Juice starts to spill over the tops of her fingers.

He backs up slowly, still holding the offending bag of Genoa that got him into this predicament. "No, beautiful. I don't. But you're glowing more and more every single day."

"Let me show you." Corinna pulls her arm back to launch the tomato at her brother. I have little doubt she'll miss as she's hurled any number of items at him.

But before this can cause Freeman Family War number 8,612 less than two weeks before Jenna's wedding, I have to intervene. I, bravely in my estimation, step in front of the missile. "Cori, everyone? Why don't I go get everyone else Genoa and we can eat while we talk about bachelorette party plans for Jenna tonight."

Actual tears fill Corinna's eyes. "You'd do that?"

"That's because she's one of us," Cassidy declares loyally.

"A Freeman," Em says with satisfaction, sending a chill that has nothing to do with the dripping tomato goo sliding down my arm on its way toward my blush-colored tee. This feeling right here is why I'll do anything; I'll give up everything.

It's because they accept and love me for who I am.

"And because Lynne is a woman. It obviously makes a difference. Thank you, Lynne. Ali knows our orders. Come on, Em. We were on with the guys about security for the wedding."

Phil looks abashed. "I'm so—"

"Save it," Holly snaps. She dashes back into her office and comes out with a roll of paper towels. Carefully, she wipes the juice from my arm upward where Corinna still has a death grip on my hand. "Come on, Cori," she cajoles her. "Lynne's going to make everything better."

Corinna's wild eyes haven't left mine. And I'm concerned because I don't see her chest moving up and down. "Corinna, breathe!" I snap.

Finally, she does. And her eyes narrow in the direction of her brother before she drops the tomato in the waiting paper towel and stomps off.

Holly, Ali, and I let out a mutual sigh of relief. "That was close," I joke.

"You have no idea. I swear since her surgery years ago, her sense of smell has increased tenfold," Phil chimes in.

Holly and Ali yell, "Shut up, Phil!" triggering my laughter.

"What's so funny?" Ali snaps.

"Nothing is ever dull here. Weren't you the one who was just saying you didn't have anything to be mad at him about?"

Ali opens and closes her mouth just as Holly bops her gently upside the head. "You jinxed all of us."

"I guess I did."

"So, Lynne. If you're going back to Genoa," Phil starts to wheedle.

But I'm already shaking my head. "No. I am not buying you anything."

He's already pleading, "It's not for me. It's for Jason. I forgot to pick up his sandwich."

Ali slaps her hand against the wall. "If, and that's a big if, Lynne gets your hubby food, we want a photo from *his* phone thanking her for it."

With a large swallow, Phil agrees.

"Fine. We'll add a Capone to the order. Now, get away from me before I have you banned from the bachelorette party," Ali snarls. Curling her finger at me, we reenter her office before she slams the door behind us. "God, I should on sheer principle. That was a serious crap thing for him to do especially to Corinna."

"Agreed it was. But could you look him in the eye at the wedding?" I might not have the same family relationships as the Freemans, but through them I've learned what I do want.

Honesty. Loyalty. Trust. No lasting relationship can withstand the test of time without those things.

"Damnit, no. Okay, fine. But can we have him come down after whatever you have planned on Thursday?"

Assuring Ali this was a distinct possibility despite knowing it isn't, we resume talking about Jenna's party while Ali puts in an order online for pickup at the Freemans' favorite Italian deli in nearby Ridgefield.

4

LYNNE

"God, do you remember when Dad used to play this song to Em?" Jenna laughs as she reaches over for the stereo remote and cranks the volume up.

"Better yet, remember when you and I would pretend to be backup singers?" I toss back.

We both leap up when the refrain comes on and screech from the top of our lungs and sing into our imaginary microphones. Finn stumbles walking back in carrying two glasses of wine, wincing at the sound.

Jenna blows him a kiss. "You don't appreciate musical genius, babe."

"I do. That just wasn't even close."

I wipe tears of laughter from my eyes. "Come on, Jen. Admit it. Your father's musical talent was definitely not inherited."

"Sadly, he couldn't teach either of us how to carry a tune," Jenna agrees. "And we all know Em can't sing."

Em's curled up on one of the overstuffed couches with her legs tucked under her. "That's the truth."

"What are you all going to do if Brendan pulls you up onstage during the wedding reception?" Jake Madison strides into the room with three more glasses of wine. Serving Em first, he hands me the next one before grabbing the remote and reducing the volume on the speakers.

"Cry because I'm being humiliated. Then beat him. Then cry," I say immediately. I frown. "Then again, I expect I'll be doing a lot of that all day, so I might as well just beat Brendan while crying. Why stop in between?"

Em, who had been taking a sip of wine, spits it right back into her glass. Jake runs his hand over his wife's hair. "I'm so glad you learned mouth control."

"Only with you, babe."

"Oh, for God's sake, did you two have to have to go there?" Jenna demands. She's snuggled next to Finn looking very much like she's found the spark that's been missing from her for years.

"You're going to be married, Jen," her father reminds her.

"Yeah, but you're my dad. I don't need to hear about your sex life," she counters.

Jake opens his mouth and promptly receives an elbow to the gut from his wife. He glares at her, but she tips her head back and just brushes a kiss under his jaw, twining her fingers with his. I let out a sigh.

"What is it, Lynne?" Finn asks.

"That's what I wish for both of you, for myself," I admit, nodding at Em and Jake.

"What do you mean?" Jake asks, as his fingers tangle naturally in Em's curls.

I think carefully before selecting my words. "Tangible happiness."

Em laughs softly. "Oh, Lynne. I only hope when it's your time to take the fall, you don't have to go through what we did."

Stubbornly, I insist, "If it brings me the kind of love you have—that all of you have—isn't it worth it?"

"When it's with the right person, yes. But along the way, there can be such feelings of despair you feel no one will understand."

"There's pain and loneliness where you feel like you're going to drown inside your own heartbeat," Jenna interjects.

"Nights where you feel like you can't breathe wondering where the other part of your soul is," Finn murmurs.

"It's a driving force that takes over your every thought, every movement, Lynne." Jake leans forward and puts his glass down with a clink. "And it gets harder the longer you stay in it."

Three other heads nod with his assessment.

Mulling over their words, I take a sip of wine. "Love is the dance everyone wants to be on the floor for once the music starts, but how many people have the stamina to finish until the end of the song?"

Finn's eyes widen comically. "I always knew you were an extraordinarily brilliant student, Lynne, but that's profound." His silver eyes are twinkling at me.

"Listen, Professor O'Hell Yes—"

Jake chokes on his drink before wheezing. Em merely reaches up and pats him on the back.

"—at least I have the good sense to be open to love," I declare.

Wrapping an arm around Jenna, he says, "I can't wait to have an up-close and personal seat for when this happens."

I roll my eyes. Pushing to my feet, I wander around the room and reach the wall collage of Em's sketches. The montage centered around a sketch of her aunt Dee—the woman who helped raise her —Cassidy, and Phil has grown over the years. My eyes home in on the ones from the summer we met in Nantucket. Lifting my glass to my lips, I momentarily get lost in the memories. "I still have the first sketch you ever did of me framed, Em."

"Oh, honey." Em slips out from under Jake's arm and moves to stand next to me. Wrapping an arm around my waist, she leans her head against mine. "Do you remember what I told you?"

I nod even as I swallow another sip of wine to prevent the burn behind my eyes from turning into tears. Tossing my short glossy hair, I recall exactly what Em told me as we overlooked the Atlantic. "You are that beautiful. Remember that. Fashion doesn't change that."

"Do you remember my agreeing, Lynne?" Jake recalls.

"I do." I toss him a warm smile. "For a long time, it was a toss-up who I had a bigger crush on, you or Brendan."

Jake roars with laughter. "Please be sure to mention that to him."

"Jake," Em scolds.

I grin at Jenna, who's sputtering with laughter into her wine. Then as Em squeezes my shoulder and makes to move away, I reach up and stop her. "I've never had a chance to say this. I hope you all will give me a moment to."

"What's that?"

Every eye is focused on me. I twirl the stem of my glass. Ruby-red liquid swirls up the wider part of the bowl. "It's not a secret to anyone hear how my family treated me. They berated me for being overweight. It was really Jenna and Jake, then Em, and the extended Freeman family who helped me transform from the anxiety-ridden girl into who I am today." I take a deep drink before joking, "Now, if a miracle would just happen and I found a love like all of you have."

Em reaches over and presses her hand against my cheek. "All we did was support you, Lynne. You did all of the work."

"You have no idea how many nights I wished I was a real member of this family," I rasp.

"And who says you aren't?" Jake asks.

I have no response to that. But I almost fall over in shock when it's Finn who replies to the tail end of my earlier statement about my family. "You're a brilliant woman, Lynne. You've obviously learned not all families are the same."

"Of course. Neither are people. Men on the other hand..." I shrug. "Let's just say I've had unfortunate taste."

"Deplorable if they treated you poorly. But let's look at an example. Take my cousin Rosie."

"Back in class, are we, Finn?" I inquire.

He shoots me the stern look I earned on more than one occasion. "There's no assignment after tonight's lesson, Ms. Bradbury."

Jenna mutters beneath her breath. I bite my lip to hold in my laughter, remembering the night when the blonde knockout threw herself in Finn's arms and kissed him soundly on the lips in front of Jenna right after she and Finn first reunited when they were in a pub in Dublin. Jenna almost clawed the other woman's eyes out before finding out they were related.

Not missing Jenna's reaction, Finn rolls his eyes. "Even if she wasn't my cousin, she wouldn't be my type. Despite how lovely she is, she's a fecking hurricane causing destruction wherever she goes."

"And your point is what, Finn?" I demand.

"That despite rumors to the contrary, men—at least good men—look beyond what's on the surface to the woman beneath. They want someone they can come home to and talk to, curl up with, and lay their worries upon. Their woman should be a safe haven for their hearts," Finn concludes.

I'm frozen until Jake asks, "And that's all you're doing with my daughter. Right, Finn? Those noises I heard the other night were just the house settling?"

"*Póg mo thóin*," he growls at Jake.

Jake just raises a brow and tsks at him.

"Do I even want to know what Prof...damnit! Finn. Finn, Finn, Finn, just said to your father?" I ask Jenna, who's wiping her eyes from laughter. Em's shaking next to me.

"Sure. He just told my dad to kiss his..." But before she can finish the statement, Finn's lowered his mouth to hers to stop the insulting words from escaping.

I grin at Finn's very effective technique for shutting up my best friend.

"Lynne." Em takes my hand. "Just trust your heart when the time comes for you to get on that dance floor you mentioned. It will guide you through the correct steps." Then, she pulls me into her arms for a long hug, giving me the understanding I've never had from my biological family but that the Freemans have so readily offered.

And without a doubt, I'd do anything for them to repay them for it. Even if that means humiliating myself with Jenna's cousin by marriage, Brendan Blake, onstage at her wedding.

Because that's what family does. In our hearts, we know there's not a damn thing we won't do for each other.

5

MARCO

"I think you two are going to have another hit on your hands with *Corps*."

Evangeline Brogan tosses her glossy brown hair over her shoulder before touching her glass of Gatorade to my brother's. "That's if the dance numbers don't kill me first. Christ, every opening night makes me miss Mom and Veronica more than ever." Quickly, she takes a sip, puts her glass down, and buries her head into her husband's shoulder.

Monty runs a hand up and down her back. "Shh, babe. It's okay. You know they were both right there with you when you flubbed your fouettés at the end of the first act."

I lean forward and rest my lips against the tips of my fingers so Evangeline doesn't spot my smile. Unfortunately, Simon isn't quite so quick. His bark of laughter escapes, earning him a smack upside his head from his wife, Evangeline's half sister, Bristol Brogan.

"You take that back, Montague Parrish! My fouettés were perfect!" she snaps.

He holds up his hands and wiggles it back and forth as if to say, *Meh*. Evangeline slaps his hand down. "Don't. You. Dare. I want to see your ass up on that stage under the burning lights en pointe. Then you can tell me who flubbed what." She stands up and storms off to their kitchen.

Monty winks at the rest of us before following her. "She'll stew on that for a bit instead of crying which she'll hate more."

After Monty walks away to go after Evangeline, Bristol leans over and covers my hand. "They're good. He's great."

"That's all I need to hear." Monty and Evangeline's courtship was riddled with drama that makes the acting she and Simon do on Broadway tame by comparison. Fortunately, what could have broken both of them actually fused their hearts together.

They're so different than Simon and Bristol. My baby brother is almost a social comedian. When I look at him, it's almost like looking in a mirror of myself. Before our mother's death when I had to worry about money. Before I used myself for the unthinkable. That's when I swore I'd have enough money no one I loved would ever have to worry again.

I take a long drink to bury the memories of those long-ago days in France. I'm no longer that man, I remind myself.

God, it's been thirteen years since I packed my bags to move to the US under a work visa. So much has changed in that time. From the slums of the city to the Upper West Side. Washing dishes during the day to augment the paltry salary I earned at Club so I could learn the ropes, not wanting to touch my savings that I sacrificed my soul for. I can almost forget what those months were like while I spent time scouting locations in the heart of Manhattan. I'd come close to signing a lease and then would second-guess myself.

And then Louie came to work at Club with me. And in the big man, I found a kindred spirit.

We were both seeking redemption.

While Simon was treading the boards in London, already beginning to make a name for himself at a young age, I was exposed to more of the city as my friendship with Louie grew. He's the one who taught me that there was life, even exclusivity, beyond Manhattan. "Think bigger, Marco. You want a club where patrons fly in on their private jets into Westchester."

And even though I laughed at him at the time, I bought an abandoned warehouse on the outskirts of the city in Fort Washington. It was a visual eyesore, but even as I signed away a good portion of my savings, I figured I could repair the outside and flip it to get something downtown.

Louie's sister worked for a satellite radio company. I thought he was crazy to suggest using some of our precious marketing budget to advertise nationally. That was until he said, "My pa always told me you dress for the job you want, Marco. You want this club to be the most exclusive one on the East Coast? Then that's how we behave from the moment we open the doors."

The first weekend, we broke even.

The second, we made a profit of sixty dollars.

By the middle of the third week, I invested that sixty dollars to buy stationery to send handwritten notes to some of the most influential people in New York advising them I'd waive their five-hundred-dollar cover charge and drinks for the evening if they presented this invite at the door.

They came back on their own the fourth week.

Each year, I've increased Louie's percentage of the business. He might sit in front checking people off the VIP list, but that's because he enjoys the energy from the people before they walk in. The reality is, he owns almost as much of Redemption as I do.

And business is very good.

With that, I face my sister-in-law and ask, "So, how does it feel to be working on your own?"

Bristol smiles. "Better now."

I frown. "You weren't happy?"

She shakes her head. "There was too much work for just me. But I landed a jewel of an employee about six months ago."

"Oh? Simon didn't mention it."

"That's because he's too busy being laughed at by Stef in tights," Evangeline taunts as she comes back into the room. "Apparently his jetés were fairly pathetic."

Simon growls from where he's singing a bedtime song to my nephew. But instead of rising to the bait, he just returns to singing.

Bristol's smile is tender. It's hard to imagine her as the woman who's been declared "Queen of Wall Street." "So, this woman helps, n'est-ce pas?"

"Incredibly so." Bristol faces me and launches into a diatribe about how her new employee has traveled the world securing new clients so Bristol herself didn't need to. "In addition, she's a financial wizard herself."

"Impressive. Are you going to let her lose on my portfolio?" I tease, already knowing her answer.

"Of course. I've given up on trying to make you bend to my will."

"What about Ev's?" I name Evangeline's father—a software billionaire—just to get a rise out of her.

"Don't be daft, Marco." Bristol rolls her eyes. "Ev listens to me."

Simon walks by with Alex cradled to his chest. "Yeah, Marco. Don't be daft."

"If you didn't have my nephew in your arms, I'd show you who's the foolish one," I challenge him. Just because I'm pushing forty doesn't mean I couldn't take him.

Simon's eyes glitter with excitement just the way they did when we were boys romping around the schoolyard. Before our lives changed; before everything changed. Then he leans down and kisses his son's head. "Give me a few and I'll take you up on it."

"You should work on your jetés instead before Stef makes you do so in rehearsal tomorrow," Evangeline purrs.

Everyone barks out a laugh except my brother. His lips just curve evilly. "Well, since we know you can't stand on one leg and twirl…"

"You fiend!" she yells.

"And they're off." Monty takes a long drink of coffee. Looking at Bristol, he asks, "Do your neighbors mind loud noises?"

"I don't think so. Why?"

"Because I have a feeling they're going to redo the performance live."

Since Simon comes out of Alex's room singing the opening number to *Corps*, I suspect Monty's right.

Years ago, I wouldn't have wished my life on anyone. The only thing I could do to forget the agony I lived in day after day was dance. But as my family argues through song and dance, I consider myself blessed. I may never have a woman like Evangeline or Bristol as my own because of the choices I made, but having them as a part of my family is just as important.

6
___

MARCO

The spotlights are throwing the lights against the strategically placed crystal chandeliers along with the deep pulsating beat. The mulberry crushed-velvet-lined walls which temper the sound also steal the flickering lights out of thin air. Bodies on the dance floor twist and sway in time with the throbbing of the music.

Leaning against a pillar, I take a pull from a bottle of water. I suppose I could wait for them with Louie, but I don't feel like dealing with all the other people coming and going. Tonight's going to be fun, I remind myself. It's rare I allow Redemption to be used for an event like this. But it's special.

All of the Freemans are.

It's incredible how much their own history reminds me of aspects of my own. *Non*, I correct myself. Their past was forced on them. My dark path was chosen. A means to an end.

And it led me here.

I feel a hand on my shoulder. It's unmistakable. I spin around and take in Corinna's slightly flushed face. Her second pregnancy agrees with her. When I spread my arms wide, she immediately moves into them. "Ah, *ma chère amie*, you look beautiful as always."

She tips her face back for a kiss, which I bestow on both cheeks. Her eyes are dancing. "You don't know how much I—we"—she rubs her hand over her baby bump— "want to go down on the dance floor."

I toss back my head and laugh. Bending down so she can hear me, I say into her ear, "I think not. Colby texted me earlier to keep a strict eye on you. Something about prohibiting table dancing?"

Corinna pouts prettily. "He's no fun at all."

"Because he loves you and wants you safe. Such a horror." I leave my arm around Corinna's shoulders as I set about welcoming the rest of the party with her. "Welcome to Redemption, ladies."

Corinna's slightly older sister Ali and slightly younger sister Holly are already attracting more than their fair share of male attention. With a quick flick of my eyes, I motion to the guards I have nearby. The woman in this group will be protected all night.

Cassidy steps forward and holds out her hand. I lift it to my lips. "Ah, Cassidy. It is always so good to see you."

She smiles before stepping forward to lay her cheek against mine. "Thank you for hosting us, Marco. It is incredibly sweet."

I'm taken aback as I've been called many things, but sweet isn't one of them. Cassidy laughs at the look on my face as she moves back. Em waves her hello as she attempts to control Phil. I recognize Jenna's mother, Michelle, from the one time I met her at the farm after Jenna's graduation. I smile at her in greeting. That leaves the guest of honor and— "Who's the woman with Jenna?" I lean down to ask Corinna.

She frowns up at me before dragging me through her siblings. As we approach, my stomach twists. Maybe it's because I've become friends with the Freemans, but I'm wary about meeting the curvy brunette. But before I can slip into my professional persona, Jenna's throwing herself into my arms. "Thank you so much for having us, Marco!"

Her face is alight with undiluted happiness. I brush a kiss across her forehead. "Be happy, *ma petite*."

"I will." Stepping back, she drags me forward a bit before raising her voice. "I don't know how the two of you have never met considering how often you both have been to the farm, but Lynne Bradbury, this is the one and only Marco Houde. Marco, my best friend, Lynne."

I'm completely unprepared for the kick to my stomach when I take Lynne's extended hand. Her dark lashes lift and reveal the most perfect azure eyes I've ever seen. "*Bonsoir, Mademoiselle Bradbury.*"

"*Comment allez-vous, Monsieur Houde? Merci de nous accueillir ce soir.*" I'm startled to hear my own tongue spoken back to me with such precision.

"You're welcome," I answer in English in response to her thanking me for hosting the group that evening. Not letting her hand go, I tilt my head before asking inanely, "You speak French?"

"*Un peu.* I've actually picked up a little bit of a number of languages for my work."

I'm about to ask her what she does, when I realize there's a stillness surrounding us despite the perpetual motion of the club at any given time. After giving her hand a gentle squeeze, I let it go. I gesture broadly. "Let me escort all of you to your section for this evening." With a nod to one of the guards, he steps in front of the group. "If you will all follow Pierre."

Jenna's strutting as she takes the lead, with Em and Michelle not far behind. I smile as both ladies surreptitiously dab under their eyes. It takes strong women to share the love of a daughter. And Jenna's relationship with her mother was strained until Em came into her life. Phil holds out an arm for Cassidy, whose hips are swaying to the beat as well. Holly and Ali make no pretense about not dancing. They're tangoing down the aisle with exceptional style. But it's the last woman who precedes me that grabs my attention.

Lynne Bradbury.

Her one-shouldered asymmetrical dress is more modest and somehow sexier than most of the women here. It's cut low enough in the back her creamy skin is on display in direct contrast to her wedge-cut dark hair. And as her legs shift back and forth, appearing longer in the pencil-thin sandals she's wearing, her curvaceous hips sway beneath her dress. And just then rows of crystal beads are caught by a spotlight, sending a shower of light everywhere.

This woman is dangerous. And having spoken with her for just the briefest of moments, I can tell she's never been touched by the atrocities my life was riddled with. In other words, I need to stay far away from her for her own good despite what my body's telling me.

But it doesn't help when Corinna slips her hand in the crook of my arm and yells, "Well, this is interesting."

I lock my jaw but don't say anything.

It might be interesting, but it can't be anything. Not for a night, not ever.

I thought it might be possible for two broken souls to come together. Once. Many years ago. Since then, I've realized it's better I remain alone. Then nothing I need to redeem myself for can taint another individual.

Especially a woman who has a whole future ahead of her.

7

LYNNE

As I sip a drink in the VIP area, my lips curve in contemplation as Jenna throws down with Ali. She has no idea of the rest of the guest list due to arrive shortly. "I hope all of this works out without the place being torn to the ground," I worry aloud.

"*Pardon, mademoiselle?*" Christ, Marco Houde's voice coming at me from behind sends shivers up my spine.

Spinning around, I find myself almost eye level with Marco's obsidian eyes. Damn, this man is absolutely gorgeous. My fist at my side clenches slightly. Leaning forward, I rephrase. "I hope Jenna likes the last part of her surprise. And that the media doesn't find out."

"Ah. That isn't something you need to concern yourself about, Ms. Bradbury..."

"Lynne," I correct him automatically. I know Marco's nearing forty, but he easily could pass for a much younger man. His olive-toned face is almost free of lines, either due to excellent genetics or a remarkable plastic surgeon. Though I suspect the former because of the fan lines that crinkle as he greets everyone. In the dim lighting of the club, it's hard to tell.

But wow. Despite the warnings in the limo, no one had truly prepared me for the sexual impact of Marco Houde. The sheer force of will it took for me to maintain a grip on his hand as currents of electric shock ran through my system were almost more than I could bear. *How does a man like that live with the sheer volume of magnetism running through him all the time?* I wonder. When he doesn't say anything, my heart begins to beat in that long-forgotten, painful thrum I thought I was over. My eyes break away from his and turn to scan the scantily clad figures around the club before once again taking in my friends, my family, before returning to his. "Unless you find it difficult to be polite to unattractive women, Mr. Houde. Don't worry, I've had that problem before."

"*Pardon?*" He looks like he wants to say more, but there's a stir at the front of the VIP section.

I place my drink down and stride forward, because even though she's wearing a full cloak, I recognize the woman beneath it. She flings it off, revealing a plum-colored dress Em made for her and hair the same shade as Jenna's.

Jenna trips in her excitement, knocking into Ali. "Dani! What are you doing here?" Ali catches her with a huge smile on her face.

I laugh. "Surprise! Did you think we all weren't coming?"

Jenna runs into her cousin's arms. As she does, I feel an arm slide around my waist. Twisting, I smile at Corinna. "You're amazing, Lynne. And I'm apparently not the only one who's noticing." Corinna discreetly nods in the direction where I left Marco.

I snort derisively. "Please. That man definitely does not care for me. Then again, there are few who do."

Much to my surprise, she slaps my ass. I jump a bit. "Jeez, Cori. What the hell was that for?"

"For putting yourself down. You know damn well there are men who love curves. Hello, Colby?" She points at her own protruding stomach.

"I knew I should have totally plied my sixteen-year-old wiles on your man," I joke.

"God, do you remember the day he answered that call Em made from the beach?" Cori reminisces.

"Oh yeah," I sigh happily.

The two of us hold in our laughter for about point two seconds before we're holding each other up. I lean over and rest my head against hers, the comfort of long friendship allowing me to place a hand against her stomach. The baby inside is having as much fun as the rest of the Freemans are. Wickedly, I wonder since it's a girl if she'll dance on tables the way her mama loves to. "I'm so glad we're here, but..."

"But what?" There's concern in Cori's voice.

"I don't fit in. Unless I'm behind a desk crunching numbers, I never really feel like I do," I say simply. "God, it feels good to tell someone that."

"Boy, do I understand that feeling," Cori says with feeling.

"I grew up privileged, yes." I wait for Cori's acknowledgement before continuing. "But with the way my parents constantly shredded my ego because I didn't conform to their image of how a Bradbury should act or how a Bradbury should look, there are parts of me that will always be scarred."

"And Marco said something that brought this back?" she presses.

Mimicking his voice, I repeat, *That isn't something you need to concern yourself about, Ms. Bradbury,* before giving a derisive snort. "Please, Cori. Part of my job is to observe and catalogue details. It's what makes me so damn good at my job. He doesn't know Michelle, but still addresses her by her first name. Me? I obviously repulse him." Before Corinna can defend her friend, I hold up a hand. "I just need a few minutes to get myself together. Tonight is about Jenna."

Turning away, I hear Corinna call out, "Where are you going?"

"I need to feel free for a few minutes, that's all. Trust me, no one will miss me."

Then slipping out of the VIP section, I spy the stairs leading down to the dance floor. If there's one thing I learned about my time in all the London Underground club scene, it's that I know how to dance.

And I sure as hell don't need anyone else to do it.

BY THE TIME the third song has ended, I've lost my inhibitions. I've forgotten about how I look and am concentrating solely on how I feel.

And right now, that's damn good.

Somewhere between slipping out of the VIP section and edging my way onto the dance floor downstairs, each step has transported me back to the clubs in London where all that matters is the dance. I no longer feel less because of who I am, but I gather strength as the music hits me from all sides, filling that missing piece of my soul.

My hair flips as I straighten my arms before whirling them over my head. Hip roll punctuated with a few elbow thrusts at chest level, I swivel on the balls of my feet before curling into a tight ball and exploding into a small leap. I don't feel the pinch in my four-inch heels as they slide across the maple-colored engineered floors.

I feel freedom.

Twirling in a tight circle, I kick out my heel, bend at the waist, right elbow to left knee, then reverse. I drag my hand up to my hair, run it through before widening my step, a quick ball change in that position, and grinding myself down until my knee touches the floor. Hold, then back up halfway before a quick hip roll, wrapping my arm around my body as the spotlight bounces off me.

Wolf whistles and catcalls start, but I don't pay any attention. I'm not dancing for whomever is making the noise; I'm dancing for me. Always for me.

I draw my fingers up the leg of my dress that Em shortened, suddenly grateful for the freedom of movement, the inhibition. My shoulders shrug up and down as I move my hands side to side, flicking the lower beading back and forth, giving the impression of sensuality, of hands behind me.

And that's when I realize there's actually someone behind me.

A hand slides around my midriff and pulls me against a hard body. "Let's see how you dance with a partner, *mon étoile*." Marco's dark voice is right against my ear.

I can't help the involuntary shudder that racks through me. But still, I'm not about to let this condescending jerk know that. "I can partner just fine. What about you?" I say archly.

His eyes narrow briefly before he spins me out and then yanks me back against his body.

Hard.

8

MARCO

"You like her," Corinna declares.

"I don't have time for this, Cori. I'm working." I try to dismiss her, but I should know better. Corinna Freeman-Hunt is so determined to see me happy, she's not about to let a little thing like a VIP party stand in the way of making that happen.

She merely rolls her eyes. "Please. Do you see my family? Do they look like they need anything?"

With a sigh, I capitulate. There's no way I'm getting out of this conversation. Briefly I scan the VIP area but don't see the lovely Lynne anywhere. Likely she just stepped out to use *la toilette*. "She's... intriguing." And before Corinna can probe any further, I add on, "And way too young and good for a man like me."

Corinna's eyes start to spike brown through the gold. I groan, "*Merde*. What did I say?"

"You do realize Jenna's fiancé is only a year younger than you?" Corinna's words almost knock me off my feet.

"Seriously?"

"Why does age matter when it comes to love? For that matter, why does sex, skin, or the type of sex you're having? Isn't that really between the people involved? Isn't it up to the people who love you best to accept and love you anyway?"

"Well, yes."

"Then don't use that as an excuse." Corinna pokes her finger in my chest. "You forget, I *know* you. And you were an ass."

I pull back, affronted. "I was not."

"Then explain why you're singling her out from the rest of us?" Corinna demands. She nods over to where Michelle is laughing with Em. "You gave Jenna's mother—a woman you've met once—a less formal greeting. And I know you. That's not who you are, At least, not here."

I argue, "I was perfectly polite."

Corinna scoffs at me. "Right. The enticing and mysterious Marco Houde greets a woman—any woman—with reserved politeness in Redemption. Tell me, does this mean the next time I come here, will the club be under renovation to become a Regency-era tearoom?"

I shudder at the very thought. "Please. You're imagining things."

"*That isn't something you need to concern yourself about, Ms. Bradbury,*" Corinna mimics me.

I flush hotly. "The only way you know that is if she told you."

"Call it concern when I saw a discontent friend amid what should have been a joyous occasion. Lynne's smart. She recognizes there's something you don't like about her. Unfortunately, she's associated your behavior with her past." With that, Corinna moves away.

Embarrassment cascades over me. Quickly, I do my job and keep an eye on the restroom in the VIP section for Lynne to come out. I need to make amends, and quickly.

That's when I hear Jenna shout. "Damn! How do we get down to the dance floor? I want to see my bestie shake it like that up close!"

The dance floor? That can't be right. But I slip a small pair of binoculars I keep in my pocket out and see just what Jenna does from the front of the VIP section—Lynne's shapely limbs moving sensuously to the pulsating beat.

No. Fucking. Way. There's no protection down there. That delectable woman will be fair game.

Tossing the binoculars on the counter, I pull out my cell and order Louie to the VIP section immediately. After he confirms he's on his way, I slip out the back. I sneer when I do because the guard I engaged to protect the hidden entrance is talking to one of the patrons instead. With an audible growl, I hurry past. I'll deal with that later. I have to get down to the dance floor first. I'm riding the edge of a feeling I've never experienced.

To stake a claim.

As I careen down the stairs, I send a text to the DJ in the booth. I push my way through the crowd just as a Sia song begins to play.

And I witness why dance is poetry in motion.

Lynne's lost in the music, her eyes closed as her hands chase the air before touching skin that's so translucent I wonder if it will bruise when I take her in my arms for the rest of the dance. Moving forward, I place my hands on my hips and wait for the perfect moment to intersect our bodies.

When I do, a gasp of air releases from her lips. I want to drink it in. Instead, I drop my head until my lips are right next to her ear. "Let's see how you dance with a partner, *mon étoile*." My star. Because watching her on the dance floor, that's what she reminds me of—something I'll be burned by if I touch, but I can't help reaching for.

I feel the shudder that racks through her. Her impudence amuses me when she declares, "I can partner just fine. What about you?"

Instead of responding, I just spin her out and then pull her back against my body until we're pressed together face-to-face from shoulder to thigh.

Holding on to one of her hands, my other drops to her hip as I begin to salsa with her. It's such a wicked dance, even in its most basic form. "You dance remarkably well, Ms. Bradbury." I formalize her name just to see what she does.

I'm shocked when she stills and begins to pull away. "*Non*, Lynne."

Her eyes narrow. "You don't get to tell me what to do, Mr. Houde."

"Fine. Then be angry with me, but never walk away from the dance floor." I squat down in front of her and slide my hands up the back of her legs, sending her trembling. "Do you want to walk away now?" I challenge her.

"I want to murder you right now," she hisses.

"Why?"

"Because this damn dress doesn't allow for panties, and that little move..." Suddenly she's flushing while I absorb the impact of her words. "Let's just finish this so we can go back and pretend to be nice for our friends. Especially since they're all watching."

"What?" But as Lynne jerks her chin up, I follow the direction and find every member of the VIP section has spilled out to the balcony to witness my fumbling with Lynne. Instead of finding Lynne embarrassed, I find her dancing in her own world.

As Lynne executes a bend, raising the hemline of her dress dangerously high, I get behind her and wrap my arms around her waist. Sliding my hand up between her plump breasts and around her jaw, I twist it until she faces mine as I bring her to a standing position. "One thing you'll learn about me, *mon étoile*, is that you'll never fake anything."

The black of her pupils almost eclipse the blue before her lashes lower. "Sorry, Marco. I'm the kind of woman that requires proof."

I bend my knees and bring us both down into a squat, swaying. Her hands grab my outer thighs for balance. "I'd much rather you grab onto my ass, darling."

"I'm not your darling," she argues as we regain our standing position.

I trail my lips from her shoulder to her ear before whispering, "Not yet. But that's for later. Right now, just dance." Then I spin her out again to the roar of the club.

9

LYNNE

I don't know how long I remain on the dance floor with Marco, but it's still too soon when he escorts me up the stairs back to the VIP section. As we both enter the back door, he growls to the abashed guard, "I'll speak with you later," receiving only a nod in reply.

Just as he's about to open the door, I touch his arm briefly. "Thank you."

His face darkens as he gets closer to me. "For what?" I open my mouth, but his finger brushes up against my lower lip. "*Mon étoile*, it is I who should be thanking you."

"For what?" I repeat his question back to him.

His lips quirk for just a moment. "For permitting me to dance with you after my earlier behavior. I've removed the stick from my ass."

I burst out laughing. "I wouldn't go quite that far."

His finger traces down my neck until it rests over the neckline of my dress. There's no way Marco can't feel the erratic beat beneath it. "But I hurt this, *non*?"

"I'm used to it," I say, but his face darkens further.

"You shouldn't be."

"That's just the way things are for a woman like me, Marco." He opens his mouth to argue, but I forestall him by reaching up and brushing my lips beneath his jaw. "Thank you for taking that away for a little while."

Slipping around him, I reach around him and open the door.

"Lynne." My name on his tongue causes me to pause.

Turning around to face him, I ask, "Yes?"

"We're not done yet." Then Marco starts to walk in the opposite direction of the VIP area. The guard I slipped past before follows him. The behemoth of a man with dark skin, a great smile, and a gold tooth who checked us in at the front door takes his place.

"I'm the kind of girl a man forgets. So, thanks for everything." Without waiting to see where they disappear to, I reenter the VIP lounge to applause.

Ali demands, "Where did you learn to dance like that?"

"Can you teach us?" Cassidy begs eagerly.

"Girl, was there a pole-dancing class involved..." The question is from Phil, of course.

Dani shoves Jenna right into Em and her mother. Phil uprights them both so they don't topple on their heels. "Can you dance like that, Miss Thing?"

Jenna shakes her head sadly. "It's pathetic when I try. Lynne took me to a club in London, and I was in shock. That's why I said you all needed to *see*."

Holly's humming happily while looking at her phone. Uh-oh. "Holly, I thought they said no photography," I demand.

"I'm not the one who took it. Louie did. He just sent it to me," she explains.

I open my mouth and close it before demanding, "Well, why didn't he take any pictures of all of you?"

"Oh, I asked him to do that," Corinna chimes in from behind me. She holds out a martini, which I gladly take a large swig of. "Trust me, Holly has enough ammo to make T-shirts for all of us in time for the holidays."

"Great. Perfect." Then I giggle. "How bad was it, really?"

"Truth?" Jenna asks.

"Always."

"I'm pretty certain the rest of my aunts are going to be knocked up by the end of the night."

I choke on my drink. "What?" I yell.

Dani raises her hand. "Me too, and Brendan is going to be in shock. That might have been the hottest thing I've ever seen in my life. It was so damn raw, I thought I was going to orgasm right here."

"Yeah, well." With everyone's eyes on me, I turn to Em and glare at her. "I'm royally pissed at you, Em."

"Why's that?" Her confusion shows behind her glasses.

Em's just taken a sip of her drink when I yell, "You try dancing with that man with no panties on!"

She immediately turns and spits her drink into her brother's face. Phil sighs before reaching in his pocket for his handkerchief. "This is the reason I wore all black tonight," he explains.

"Like that would have stopped Em," Cassidy chastises.

"True. If anything, you likely would have been a target well before now, Uncle Phil. Hey, we haven't danced yet," Jenna complains.

"Then come here, darling." Proving he's got plenty of moves of his own, Phil pulls his niece by marriage into his arms and dips her backward. "While we can't come close to Lynne and her man, we can try to hold our own."

I open and close my mouth like a fish.

Corinna comes up next to me. "It totally sucks, doesn't it?" she sympathizes.

"What? The part where I love all of you despite there being obvious mental deficiencies?"

Corinna lets out a husky laugh. "Yep. I hate to break it to you, but apparently it's environmental, not genetic. So, when you have kids, they'll be just as crazy."

"You're assuming a man will want me enough to have babies with me, Cori."

Her eyebrow wings upward. "Do I need to go get Holly's phone?"

"He danced with me. He's likely danced with a million woman. Look at where we are. I want a man who sees me, Cori. I want what all of you have."

"And you don't think that could happen with Marco?"

"Maybe it could. But why would he want it to happen with me when he could have any one of the women who come into Redemption night after night? I'm an aberration—an anomaly outside the standard deviation to use a term from work. By tomorrow, I'll be long forgotten."

"Do you have a kill list?" Corinna asks suddenly.

"A what?" I laugh.

"A list of people you would kill without question if you could get away with it."

"Does it include the random people who cut me off?"

Corinna waves her hand. "They're peons. Not worth the blood. No, I mean the people who you would love to see their blood spill."

Finishing my martini, I circle the air with it. "Can't say I've thought about it much."

"After the people who hurt my family, your parents are on mine."

My mouth falls open into a perfect O.

"What they did to you is abuse, Lynne. They destroyed a piece of your soul. You're a damn knockout, and it infuriates me you don't believe a man like Marco—hell, any man—would be interested in you. You were sixteen and my fiancé said you were going to grow up to be a heartbreaker." Getting as close to me as her pregnant belly allows, she whispers, "He didn't mean because of the fact you'd break our hearts believing the crap your parents spewed. You are brilliant and beautiful, Lynne Bradbury. And one day, a man is going to be damn lucky to know you love him."

Overwhelmed by her words, I flutter my hand in front of my eyes. "We can't do this now."

"We're going to do it soon," she warns me.

"Just...not right now. Okay?" Not when my emotions are spiking like Roku's stock price. Whirling around, I head straight for the bar to exchange my martini glass for champagne.

After all, we're here for a reason, and it's not to celebrate my abilities on the dance floor.

It's for a reason much more beautiful than that.

Love.

10

LYNNE

"Ugh, whose phone is ringing," Jenna complains the next morning, holding her head. "I think I might die."

"This is why we have the bachelorette party well before the wedding, darling." Dani comes bouncing into my bedroom. Obviously, the late night and early phone call didn't irritate her. "Lynne, it appears to be your phone. I missed picking it up, but it said, 'Bristol Calling.'"

"Shit. That's my boss." Rolling out of my king-size bed, I race into the bathroom to pee, splash some water on my face, and brush my teeth. When I come back out, Dani's taken residence in my bed. "You all suck."

"Sorry, not sorry." Dani hands me my phone.

Narrowing my eyes, I declare, "You realize I can probably shove your skinny ass to the middle and crawl back in after I'm done."

Dani immediately spreads her long arms and legs like a starfish.

Even as I leave the room so the two Madison women can fall back asleep, I'm simultaneously throwing up my middle finger behind me and calling Bristol back.

She immediately picks up. "I'm so sorry," she cries.

"You wouldn't be calling if it wasn't an emergency. Besides, I'm not that hungover," I joke.

"Thank God, though I don't think this particular set of clients would care all that much."

"What's up?" I head into the kitchen and slip a pod into my Keurig. Mentally, I'm blessing Ryan and Jared for letting me know one of the units in their building was up for sale. Even if it's not as posh as theirs is with rooftop access, living in the pre-war building is stunning. When I'm home to appreciate it, I think wryly.

"Alex has a fever, and Simon's at rehearsal and can't be reached."

"Just tell me what you need.

She continues as if I haven't spoken. "It's rare I can get these two to come in to discuss their portfolio. You know I wouldn't consider asking you to take a client meeting, but I'm afraid I'm contagious too. I've already had Rudy reschedule everything to be over the phone for the rest of the week, but I need you." Bristol sounds frenzied.

"It's okay. How much time do I have?" I soothe her.

"Three hours. God, Lynne, I'm so sorry. I promise I'll make this up to you."

"Don't worry about it. This is completely unavoidable. Does Rudy have the information about the account up so I can review it?"

"Yes. And if you see something you would recommend making any changes on, give me a call. I've been managing the money for RHS, LLC for so long, I may not have seen a growth opportunity."

"I will," I promise her. "Now, let me go get changed and I'll head in."

"Call for a car." I start to protest, but Bristol overrides me. "I don't want you dealing with driving the day after a bachelorette party."

"Yes, dear," I tease.

"You're precious, and not just for that brilliant mind." With that, Bristol hangs up.

I grab the steaming coffee and head back into my bedroom. Jenna pops her head up and asks, "S'everything okay?"

"I have to go in for a few hours. I'll bring food when I come back," I reassure her.

"Okeydokey." And with that, Jenna flops out like a light.

Amused, I close the door between my bed and bath, grateful my walk-in closet is off the bathroom. I pull out a deep mulberry suit, black Louboutins with a pencil-thin heel, and iridescent gray pearls I nabbed at Mikimoto the last time I was in Tokyo. Fortunately, it only takes me about forty-five minutes to get ready.

I'm shoving my laptop, iPad, and wallet in my briefcase, when Em comes stumbling out of one of my guest rooms. "Whoa, did we time warp? Where are you going looking so good?"

I walk around the counter and drop a kiss on her head. "I have to head into work for a few hours. I'll be back with food. Text me if you want anything special. I have a car waiting downstairs. Love you, Em."

"Well, since you look like you're going to take over the world, have fun doing so." She yawns before spying the Keurig. "Coffee!"

I'm laughing as I walk out the door.

AN HOUR LATER, I'm on the phone with Bristol. "Riddle me this, why are the clients afraid of a more aggressive portfolio? Are they nearing retirement?"

She laughs wearily. "Picked up on that? No, the clients have what they consider a risky investment that takes up a large portion of their capital. They want their portfolio to be fairly risk-free so they don't have to worry about their lifestyle should something else happen."

My eyes scan the screen in front of me. "We could do that and just play with a portion of the interest."

"Hmm. You mean the way you do with Ryan's money?"

"How did you know about that?" I demand.

"He told me, of course. You turned a cool million into a hundred million without losing him a dime?" I can hear her clicking her nails against the table of the doctor's waiting room. "Suggest it. Just don't be surprised if they turn you down."

"You're serious?" I'm surprised.

"Very. And Lynne..." She's about to say more, but I hear Alex's name being called. "Drat. I have to go. I'll call you later."

"Sounds good. Take care of your guys."

While I'm waiting for the client to show up, I pull up a modeling software I've used for years. "If I had even 50K..." And soon I'm lost in charting potential growth based on current market trajectories. Time flies until there's a knock at my door. "Come in," I answer absent-mindedly.

I can hear Rudy in the hall before he opens the door. "Gentlemen, as I stated, Ms. Brogan is out ill. This is her second-in-charge, Lynne Bradbury. Lynne, I'd like to introduce you to the owners of RHS, LLC. First, this is Mr. Louis Scott."

I'm almost stunned speechless when Louie, Marco's bouncer, gives me a wide smile and a wink as he takes my hand and raises it to his lips. "Good to see you looking so bright this morning, Lynne."

Rudy laughs. "I didn't realize you all knew each other. Then I'm certain you know the other client."

Then Marco's face appears over the top of Rudy's. "Bristol Brogan-Houde. Why did I never put it together?" Coming out from around the desk, I hold out my hand. "Good morning, Mr. Houde."

He covers his own shock quickly. "Good morning, Lynne. Shall we begin?"

"Certainly. Can Rudy bring either you or Mr. Scott—"

"Louie, please," Louie corrects me.

"I didn't want to presume with a client." I flash him a quick smile. "Can we get either of you gentlemen some coffee?"

Both men nod. "Lynne, do you need a refill?" Rudy offers.

"Please." As I return to the place behind my desk, I slide two thick envelopes across the table. "Gentlemen, inside those folders are your annual reports. I'd like to review them with you." Immediately they reach for them, but just as they touch them, I drop the bomb. "But when we're talking, I'd like to discuss how you could be making more with hardly any risk."

Marco's eyes fly up to mine. In them there's wariness and distrust.

Let's see what he has to say when I'm done talking.

11
MARCO

I can't focus on a single word Lynne's saying, and they're damned important words. She's flinging around numbers as if they're simple math equations, however it's millions of dollars, my safety net and Louie's in the event something ever happens to Redemption.

Neither of us have ever touched a dollar in the RHS, LLC fund. Year over year, it's increased steadily, though Bristol has practically pleaded with us to let her spread out our investments. "A little diversity won't kill you, Marco."

But I refuse to be budged. I won't be in a position where I have to beg for food, where I need to rely on someone else's largess, where a good tip makes or breaks being able to pay for rent. I recall the days where that included my brother's tuition as well. My fist clenches in my lap. No, never again. Ms. Bradbury can take Bristol's suggestions and...

"So, let's talk about my suggestion." Lynne relaxes in her chair. Based on the way Louie's smiling, he's happy right now.

I try to relax, but this is too important. "I refuse to sink large parts of our capital into any kind of fly-by-night fantasy." Part of my life revolves around creating a fantasy for people. In this, I have my feet firmly planted on the ground.

Much to my surprise, Lynne laughs. "Trust me, I understand."

"There's no way you could," I shoot back.

"Actually, when it comes to this, I do. The RHS, LLC investment plan is similar to my own."

Louie booms out a laugh. "Are you joking, Lynne?"

"Not at all." Turning, she types on her keyboard before a few pieces of paper print out. She hands them across the table. I lean forward and take it. I'm astounded to find it's her own portfolio data. "I truly believe in practicing what I preach, gentlemen."

"Are these real numbers?" I'm stunned. The voluptuous young woman in front of me is worth almost as much as I am. I glance at Louie and find his lips parted in shock.

She shrugs before holding out her hands. We both put the paper back in them and she immediately tears it into little pieces. "The reality is all I showed you were numbers on a piece of paper. What do you know about me?"

"Not a lot," I say. But I want to know more.

"Exactly." She beams at me like I'm a prize student. She types again and takes two more sheets of paper and slides them across the table. "This is just a model," she warns.

As Louie and I reach for the paper, I'm suddenly curious about what Lynne's about to propose.

And as I begin to read, I think now I know something else about her.

She's brilliant.

AN HOUR LATER, paperwork signed, Lynne is escorting me and Louie to her office door. "I'm pleased you feel confident with Bristol to try out that proposal." She offers her hand to Louie.

He ignores it and scoops her up in a hug, much like the one he gave her last night. "We believe in you, Lynne. Bristol's terrific, but she's a wolf. You complement her."

Lynne's smile reflects her joy. "Thank you. You have no idea how deeply that touches me."

"I bet your parents are awfully proud to have a daughter like you."

Lynne's head turns to the side as she forces out brightly, "Actually, Louie. My biological parents haven't spoken with me since I was eighteen. I wouldn't know if they're proud of me or not."

"What?" I burst out.

She ignores me to finish. "But since I've been pretty much adopted by the Freeman family, I can assure you that, yes, they're very proud of the success I've attained."

"Louie, would you mind meeting me out front?" I grind out.

"Sure." He slips out the door, leaving the two of us alone.

"This is what you meant last night when you said you were used to being hurt."

Lynne shrugs as if her parents' attitude means little when it's obvious it means a great deal. "Don't worry about it, Marco. I'm used to it. I rarely see them."

"Rarely?" I question.

"I might run into them the week of the wedding, but there's no avoiding that on a place as small as Nantucket. I just ignore them."

"And what do they do, *mon étoile*?"

"Nothing." I let out a sigh of relief but too soon when she softly adds, "Anymore."

"*Putain de merde!*"

Much to my surprise, Lynne holds up a finger and tsks me. "Such language."

And after brief pause, I burst out laughing. "I thought you understood beginner French?"

"Well, when you have to explain to a French count that despite your written recommendation, his decision to invest in his friend's company cost him most of his fortune, you pick up a great deal of the...local color," she explains.

I'm still chuckling when I reach for her. "Do you understand what I'm calling you?" I reel her in slowly, giving her a chance to escape. One arm bands around her hips, and the fingers of my other tangle in the ends of her hair.

Her eyes don't leave mine, but her hands find my wrists and grip. "No, I don't."

"Let's see if I can make you see them," I murmur. Then I lower my head and brush my lips against hers. Pausing, I wait to make certain I'm not going to be slapped for kissing her in her place of business.

Her hands slide farther up until they grip my biceps through my suit jacket. "Again." The words leave her mouth and enter mine on the same breath.

I don't bother to reply. I simply slant my head, my parted lips sealing over hers. My tongue flicks out to taste her lips. Between one heartbeat and the next, her lips part, giving me the access I need. Slipping inside, my tongue finds hers, then retreats, daring hers to come after mine. To my delight, it does.

Lynne twines her arms around my neck, pulling our bodies closer to one another. Now, I feel every soft ripple against my body. Everything I imagined on the dance floor last night. As her greedy fingers thread through my hair, I tighten my arms around her and pull her hips into my aroused body.

Our tongues continue to duel back and forth in this drugging, arousing kiss. I forget where we are as I begin stroking her curves through the material of her suit. It isn't until her phone rings persistently that I remember. "*Mère de Dieu?* What are we doing?"

Stepping away slightly, Lynne runs a finger beneath her lips before doing the same to mine. "I think it's called kissing," she whispers conspiratorially. "But if you're not convinced, I might be convinced to give you another demonstration." Lynne moves behind her desk and sits down.

I begin to laugh. "Minx. You seduce me with the way your body moves on a dance floor, then with your mind. What's next?"

"Since I wasn't trying to do either, be sure to let me know. I'll take notes. I'm a really good student." She picks up a pen as if to take notes.

I bend down and pick up the folder I dropped. "Is your personal number in here?"

She holds out her hand. Pulling out the card she slipped inside the folder, she writes a number on the back. "It is now."

"I'll text you. I have to work tonight," I apologize.

"And I have the family at my condo, Marco." Lynne's voice is hesitant. "There's something you should know about me."

"Oh? What's that?" I'm waiting for something truly horrible. So, my heart breaks at her next words.

"Even if you never call, that was the best kiss I've ever had. And if you don't call, don't worry. I never have any expectations." Picking up her phone, she presses a number. "Yes, Mr. Houde is ready to be escorted out. Thank you."

Within seconds, Rudy is opening the door and I'm meeting Louie in the lobby. It isn't until we're on the elevator that he asks me, "What took you so long?"

"I got her number."

Louie rolls his eyes. "It was in the folder. She gave it to both of us."

Turning to my longtime friend, I explain, "No, I was getting her number," just as the elevator doors open and I step out.

I must have stunned him because he doesn't follow me. I hear him curse as he's slapping buttons. "Are you serious?"

"I told you, I asked for her number," I remind him impatiently as we cross the lobby and out onto the busy Manhattan street.

"No, I mean about her. She's so much more than anyone I've ever watched you date."

That surprises me enough to ask, "Including Corinna?" Louie adored Corinna, treating her like a kid sister from the moment they met.

"Different. But yes. Don't screw this up, Marco." He moves forward and whistles for a cab.

An insidious thought invades my brain. What if my life's already screwed up my chances with a woman like Lynne? I shove aside the thought as I get inside the cab alongside Louie.

But all the way back to Redemption, I can't get that kiss off my mind.

12

LYNNE

"Did you seriously say we're drinking champagne?" Jenna groans while holding her head. "That's just cruel and mean after last night."

"Aw, you poor thing," Dani snickers. "Is your head hurting?"

"Must be rough," Corinna mocks. "I don't seem to recall anyone caring when it was my bachelorette party."

Phil makes a rude noise. "Please. I think we kept you drunk for a week."

Ali's scrambling around my kitchen opening cabinets, looking for the flutes, but still manages to call out, "I'm just grateful you sobered up enough that the legality of the marriage wasn't in question."

Cassidy chortles. "We stopped drinking three days in advance just for that reason, Ali."

"I still think Cori might have been buzzed," Holly calls out from behind her camera lens. Aiming it in my direction, she takes a few shots before muttering just loud enough for me to hear, "Hmm. Just celebrating a success at work?"

I flush. "Yep." That's what I told everyone when I walked in with two bottles of Cristal a little while ago and not a single bite of food.

"Uh-huh," Holly mutters as she turns the camera around to continue taking snaps of the family.

Michelle hangs up the phone from ordering a ridiculous amount of pizza and calls out, "Twenty minutes. Lynne, go change so you're comfortable."

Setting down the champagne, I head in the direction of my bedroom. "Good idea."

Just as I head down the hall, Em yells, "You should probably use a makeup wipe to remove the smeared lipstick on your face though! You really don't want that rubbing off and ruining the silk of your suit."

All the noise from my condo ceases just as I say, "Crap."

And of course, Phil's the one who calls out, "Busted! Now get changed and get back in here to tell us all about him."

Everyone bursts into gales of laughter.

Thinking for just a second, I turn around, my heels making a definitive clicking sound on the restored parquet floors. Each step I take toward the living room causes the room's volume to decrease. Once I get into view, I wipe the giddy smile from my face.

Em starts to apologize, but I just hold up a hand. Then, unable to stand it, my smile breaks free, causing my dimple to pop out. "What makes you think you don't already know him?" Then I take off for my room at a fast clip before the inquisition can truly begin.

And honestly, I do have to get my makeup off my face. Em helped me pick out this suit; I really don't want it ruined.

For the first time ever, Phil spits his drink in Em's face. "Back it up, baby cakes. Marco kissed you?"

Instead of getting mad about the drink, Em unleashes herself like a protective mother. "And why wouldn't he? Lynne's a gorgeous woman."

"Because he's closed himself off from any kind of serious relationships since that one." Phil tips his glass in Corinna's direction. "And then there's the fact Lynne's so much younger…"

Jenna throws a pizza crust at him, nailing him soundly in the face. "Care to rephrase that, Uncle Phil?" Her voice is saccharine sweet.

But I'm stuck on the Corinna comment. Twisting in her direction, I confirm, "You…and Marco?"

She rolls her golden eyes. "Years before I even started dating Colby, Lynne. Trust me when I say we're friends and there's nothing more to it."

Maybe not on her side, but is there on his? I can't prevent the concern from worming its way into my brain.

With an ease born of practice, Corinna shifts her weight to the end of the chair and stands. She walks to where I'm cuddled with Jenna and hitches her thumb. "Beat it, kid."

Jenna scrambles to get out of the way.

Corinna settles down next to me with a sigh. "Christ, I miss sitting in chairs like this. Someone's going to have to help me out of it though."

Everyone bursts into laughter, including me. Rubbing her hand over the baby, Corinna fixes me with an intent look. "Part of the reason Marco cared for me was because he felt he could trust me. You know our"—she nods around the room—"stories."

And I was honored the day I was told them. "I do."

Corinna nods. "Marco knew there were things in my past, just as I knew there were things in his—neither of which we shared with each other in the time we were together. Looking back, I think we were friends first, and becoming lovers almost was expected? Does that make sense?"

"Were you together long?" I'm curious, not angry. What right do I have to jealousy when I would have been what, in middle school when all of this happened?

"If you count the time we were friends, we were together for years." I raise my brows. Corinna laughs. "I know; it's a shock, right? Here was this prime guy, and I felt…content."

"Um, not for nothing, but he kissed me once and that's not at all what I felt. Try a raging inferno." The entire room roars once again.

Corinna reaches over and takes my hand. "Good, because that's what you're supposed to feel. And it's what I feel—for Colby."

I squeeze hers. "I love that you both found each other."

"So are we, darling. But back to Marco." Her face takes on a thoughtful cast. "We were both young, unattached, and attracted to one another. If Colby Hunt didn't exist in this universe, who knows if it would been enough to satisfy me? Maybe I would have felt that was all I deserved. But Marco knew I had feelings for Colby. And Colby has always been the only man with the key to opening up my entire heart," she concludes.

As much as I've always adored Corinna, her honesty in what could have been a very sticky situation completely disarms me. Snuggling next to her, I whisper, "You're one of the strongest women I know."

Her lips brush the top of my head. "In a room full of them, I take that as one of the highest compliments there is. Now, as both of your friends, what are you going to do next?"

Everyone leans forward, eagerly anticipating my answer.

"I gave him my number. Honestly, the next move is his," I answer.

Corinna opens her mouth, but my cell pings. I struggle to sit up. "Christ, if I need help, Corinna's going to need a crane to get out of this couch."

"Bite me, Lynne, but you speak the God's honest truth. And it'd better be soon. I have to pee."

Ali immediately jumps up from her spot on the floor. "You always have to pee."

"Like you didn't when you were pregnant?" Corinna retorts.

I make a choking sound.

Ali drops Corinna, who curses, before turning in my direction. "What's wrong, Lynne?"

Corinna falls back with a soft plop. "Ali, you suck. Lynne, what is it?"

I turn the cell phone in her direction. "I think the next move is now in my court."

Corinna reads it quickly before saying, "I really hope the couch is treated in case I have an accident." Then she tosses my phone at me before throwing her arms and legs in the air screaming, "*Yahoooooo!*"

Jenna demands, "What does it say?"

I open and close my mouth, but I can't make words come out. I can only stare at the text from the unknown number over and over.

Mon étoile, will I get to see you before you go to Jenna's wedding?

I type one word back.

Yes.

Then I help Ali evict Corinna just in time for her to make it to the bathroom. I use the time while everyone's talking to figure out where in the schedule I so carefully planned I can see Marco.

13

LYNNE

As much as hitting Fifth Avenue with the women sounds intriguing, meeting Marco for a few hours is more so. My Jag purrs as I turn into the empty parking lot of Redemption. I'm not entirely certain why Marco wants to meet here, but I'll admit to being curious to see what the inside of the club looks like during daylight hours.

I roll down the window and press in the code Marco gave to me to unlock the gate at the front entrance of the warehouse parking lot. The moment I do, my phone rings. Pressing a button on my steering wheel, I answer Marco's call. "So, I guess saying 'Surprise, I'm here' is a bit redundant?"

His sensuous laugh sends chills up my spine. "There's a camera at the gate, Lynne. Drive around the back. Park next to my car."

I scan the parking lot up ahead for any obstructions before I ask, "You realize the urge to open up and drive in all this empty space is real?"

"Later. The sweepers haven't been by yet today to check the lot."

"I like that you're a reasonable man, Marco," I decide.

"Why would I deny you the pleasure of doing something I've done many times myself?" he asks before he disconnects the call.

"Why indeed?" But I appreciate his concern as I get closer to the building and see some of the litter. Who knows what that would have done to my undercarriage? Navigating around the warehouse, I drive forward and begin to laugh. Leaning next to a car almost identical to my own is Marco dressed in an untucked black shirt and jeans.

I don't even have time to reach for my door handle before he's there, a smile playing about his lips. "I debated the convertible," he remarks offhandedly. "But I figured since I'd be parking outside, the coupe would be a better fit."

Sliding from the car, I take his hand. "And I debated the coupe, but I said screw it. I wanted what I wanted, and to hell with what anyone thought."

"An intriguing truth." He lifts my hand, and I think he's going to kiss the back of it. Instead, he lifts my wrist to his lips and presses his lips there before he leads me to one of two doors. Using his free hand, he quickly punches in a code. "I wonder what else I'll learn about you today."

"Does that go both ways?" I ask boldly.

He stills as the door buzzes. Opening it, I'm surprised to find we're stepping directly into a service elevator. "I tell no lies. Ever. But remember, the truth isn't always as elegant as a dance," Marco says quietly.

He drops my wrist to close the gate before pressing a button. The elevator jolts as we begin moving upward, and I fall, causing Marco to catch me. He grips my upper arms as he holds me against him tightly.

His face is granite in the shadows. The only movement is the light which filters in from the warehouse windows as we climb slowly in the elevator. Light, dark, my lips part with the realization. *Just like Finn accused you of having more than one persona, he has them too.* The lack of words says more than a hundred ever could about the man holding me. But before I can make a sound, the elevator comes to an abrupt stop. Marco smiles, and it's as if the minutes before didn't happen. There's warm light coming toward us. "Where are we?" I ask.

"My home. Come, I've made lunch." Marco expertly slides open the gates and reaches for my hand.

"You live above the club?" I'm dumbfounded.

He winks. "It's a great commute, *n'est-ce pas*?"

I laugh. "A lot better than some of the ones I've had to make recently, yes. Marco, this is lovely." I spin around and take in the airy space that balances the industrial feel of the warehouse with the functional feel of a home.

Marco places a hand on my back, just above the band of my jeans. I can feel the warmth of his fingers burn through the thin material of my summer shirt. "Would you like a tour first or after we eat?"

As curious as I am, that's the moment my stomach decides to betray my earlier nerves and grumble. I bite my lip. "I think this body part"—I pat the curve—"has decided for me."

"My home goes nowhere. However, we shall compromise—an appetizer? Brie en croute?"

"Yum. Is there anything I can do to help?" I follow him over to the kitchen space.

"Yes. Sit here and tell me how ill Jenna was. It will greatly amuse me." Marco pulls out the brie from the oven and places it on the counter. He transfers it expertly onto a cheese board and hands me a knife.

I slice into it. "Well, when I walked in carrying two bottles of champagne after our meeting, I thought she was going to club me with one." Sliding the warm brie onto a piece of french bread, I take a bite and moan, "So delicious."

Marco hesitates for just a moment before stalking around the counter. I'm still holding the bread when he captures my face in between his hands and presses his mouth to mine. My fingers clench around the bread in my hand as his lips taste every inch of mine. As he pulls away, he mutters, "Tastes better flavored with you, *mon étoile*."

"Whoa." I go to fan myself but find the bread stuck to the inside of my hand. Flushing hotly, I manage to stammer, "Do you have a napkin?"

"For what?"

I hold up my hand, and he throws his head back and laughs. My eyes narrow. "Shall I retaliate?" I ask sweetly.

He opens his arms. "You are welcome to try."

I slide off my stool and swing my hips as I make my way toward him. For all he's trying to keep his cool, Marco's nostrils are flaring. His arms drop to his sides. His fists clench. Holding his gaze, I get close to him...

...and reach past him for the napkin just behind him. "Thanks. As delicious as this was, it was starting to feel a bit uncomfortable." I wipe my hand before asking, "Where can I dispose of this?"

He mutters something in French I don't entirely pick up, but his frustration is evident enough my lips twitch. "Back to your question. Once the pizza was consumed, everyone felt fine."

"Everyone? The party was still going?"

"It's going on until the wedding," I confirm.

"And you gave up time with your friends to be with me?" he asks incredulously.

"I did."

"Why, Lynne? Why would you do such a thing?" Marco reaches for me, but I evade him.

Instead, I counter his question with one of my own. "Why did you kiss me?"

14

MARCO

"I don't know," I answer her honestly. I wait for her to become angry and to storm off.

But I'm surprised when she accepts the answer. "That answer works both ways, Marco. Jenna's been my best friend since I was sixteen. I'm maid of honor in her wedding. Yet, when your text came in, something pulled at me to accept." With a self-deprecating smile, she mocks herself, "Trust me, the shopping part of girls' weekend wasn't the part I was most looking forward to. It never is."

I frown. "Why not?"

"Umm, hello?" Lynne spins around in a circle as if the answer should be apparent. "Not exactly model slim over here. The sales-people often look at me pityingly. It's a rather annoying behavior I've suffered with my entire life."

Fury grabs me by the throat. "Why? Because you have curves like a woman should? You do not resemble a skinny boy in a dress? What is wrong with that?"

Her blue eyes widen. "Nothing. I'm just used to... Nothing is wrong with it."

"You're used to *les imbéciles*," I accuse.

"If that means the same thing in English as it does in French—" Lynne begins.

I interrupt. "Fools! Why are people such fools?" I'm about to go off on a tirade about the ridiculousness of "magazine beauty" when Lynne's soft voice halts me.

"Then it wasn't just men. It was my family as well." She moves around the counter to sit down before taking a piece of bread and picking up the knife.

"*Excuse-moi*?" I lean over the counter and am as close to her as when I tasted the brie off her succulent lips.

Lynne's swollen lips part, tempting me to taste them again. But when she speaks, her voice is calm. "Maybe now's a good time to explain why I'm so close to the Freemans. *All* of them." Her emphasis on the word causes my brows to raise.

I push myself to a standing position. "You have concerns about my past...association with Corinna?"

I'm ready to present to her sound reasoning why what I had with Corinna is long past—except it was still the longest relationship I had to date, my inner voice reminds me—when she knocks me on my proverbial ass by saying, "Actually, I don't. That would be fairly ridiculous since I would have been a child. Really, Marco. You were in your late twenties?"

"About that."

Lynne rolls her eyes. "Then let's be logical. I was still crushing on the poster of Brendan Blake I had on the bulletin board in my bedroom—nor had I met any of Jenna's family yet. Are you going to hold that against me since I'll see him next week? That's grossly unfair to all of us, don't you think?"

I laugh softly. "You're..."

She bristles. "Yes?"

"Remarkable. Now you have me dying of curiosity, *mon étoile.* How did you meet Jenna and the rest of the family?"

"Every summer for as long as I can remember, my family has spent the summer at their beach house on Nantucket Island," Lynne begins. I go over to the refrigerator and hold up a bottle of sparkling water. She smiles. "Yes, thank you. It was horrid. Not that being at home wasn't bad, but being at the island was even worse. I was close with the servants. I had a few acquaintances at school, but no one I'd consider a close friend."

"Where did you live the rest of the year?"

"Not far from here—Greenwich. Oh, but don't get any ideas, Marco. My parents didn't give me the same perks they gave to my older brother and sister. I didn't quite fit the mold they did as a Bradbury." She spins the heavy glass around before taking a drink.

Deciding to ask her about her more about that later, I inquire, "What was so different about that summer?"

"Jenna and her father moved in. And we both got a job at a local coffee shop."

"And it was friendship ever after?" I mock slightly.

Lynne scoffs. "Not hardly. That summer is also the same summer Em came to prepare for her first fashion show. Talk about tumultuous feelings everywhere? God, I don't know what was more insane, the emotional pain inside Em, what I now understand as the sexual tension between her and Jake, or the pain I was going through at home. Luckily, I had Jenna to talk to, then Em." She meets my eyes directly. "And then I had Corinna. I honestly think it took all of them from preventing me from doing something drastic to escape."

Suddenly uneasy, I put my glass down. "What do you mean, 'escape'?"

Lynne slides off her stool and wanders over to a framed picture Bristol gave to me on my birthday where I'm holding Alex. Simon has his arm wrapped around my shoulders. It's one of my favorites. "Imagine if someone told this baby from the time they could talk they weren't good enough, weren't smart enough. That they physically didn't meet the family standards. That they were worthless."

My temper begins to boil, but just as I'm about to say something, Lynne continues. "Then imagine they meet one person—one single person. And that person steps forward declaring they want to do something so special to help this person."

"I'd want Alex to marry that person," I growl.

Lynne laughs softly. "Sorry, but I think Finn would be angry if I stole his bride."

My mind reels. "It was Jenna?"

Lynne nods. "She wanted to become a fashion designer solely to design a fashion line that would look good on me. Can you believe it? She battled Jake every single day. And then Em came into the picture."

"What happened?" I'm captivated by the story.

"Em did two things that changed my life forever."

"Do you mind if I ask what they were?" I approach her.

"The first thing she did was draw me a picture."

"What was it of?" But I have a strong suspicion I already know the answer.

"It was of me. In the course of a conversation overlooking the ocean, the renowned Emily Freeman drew a picture of me. Before that, I only saw myself the way *they* saw me. I never saw myself the way *others* saw me. Trust me, that plus the second were both eye-openers."

"What was the second?" I reach over and brush a piece of hair off her cheek.

Lynne's hand comes up and grips my wrist. "She called Corinna on FaceTime. And by the end of the first week after that morning at the beach, they became my friends."

Good, I think savagely. My fingers tighten in her hair. "Why have you been on your own since you were eighteen, Lynne? Did something happen to your parents?"

"You could say that." Lynne pulls away and moves back toward the counter, where she takes another sip of water. I trail behind. "I'm a smart woman, Marco. I think you've figured that out already."

"I have, yes." And for a man who only finished *l'école secondaire*, her master's from the London School of Business could be quite overwhelming if I hadn't worked so damn hard for everything I have.

"Well, before I told them to keep their money and they disowned me, they said the only way I'd earn the money for my education was if I agreed to medical treatment for my weight issues. They wanted me to delay college until I could 'finally represent the Bradbury name the way it should have been.'" She folds her arms under her ample breasts.

"I hope you told them to rot in hell."

"No."

"Pity."

"What's the point?"

"The point is..."

"Nothing." My jaw slackens at her calm. "Absolutely nothing. Do you know in the last ten years how much I've changed? I've grown from being desperately miserable to finding some sort of happy. And they had nothing to do with it. The people I consider my family did. So, that brings us around to this: Why should I care that you had an affair with Corinna? Are you still in love with her?"

I contemplate the question before answering honestly. "I think a part of me always will be."

15

LYNNE

"**B**etter not let Colby hear you say that," I tease gently to let him know I understand.

"Please. Colby has had many an opportunity to take my head off over the years. I think I helped him pull his own out of his ass to get them together," Marco retorts.

Delighted, I clap my hands together as I laugh. "Phil didn't mention that part yesterday when...oops!"

"Ah, did you kiss and tell?" The upward curve of his lips takes any edge his words might imply.

"Not on purpose, I can assure you!" I respond indignantly.

Marco smile widens. "I know. That family can ferret out information better than a team of spies. You've been the target during a family dinner, I presume?"

"Lord, I think Ali's picking up interrogation techniques from Keene! I can only imagine when Kalie and the twins start dating. Forget Keene being overprotective—Ali's going to neuter the dates first!" We both laugh.

Marco reaches over and runs his thumb over the apple of my cheek. "I'm surprised we've never met before the other night. I've been to the farm many times. Now hearing how close you are to the family, I assume it is the same for you, *n'est-ce pas?*"

"Every time I can," I confirm. "I had the same thought on the ride to the club when the family was making connections before I realized it was likely because I was traveling so much—first for Ryan, then for Bristol."

A timer dings, interrupting our introspection. "Are you hungry yet?" Marco moves over to the oven.

"Would I be terribly rude if I say not really? I did a number on the brie." But my mouth can't help but water over the spatchcock chicken he places on the burner.

"Then how about the tour before we eat?" he suggests.

"That sounds like a great plan." Standing, I wait for him to lead.

I won't lie and say I don't feel a flip in my stomach when he takes my hand to guide the way.

WE'RE SITTING down on the couch with a meal of chicken and salad having completed the tour when Marco asks about my space in Tribeca. I swallow a bite of the crispy-skinned chicken before answering. "A similar feeling to this but obviously not as spacious."

He smirks. "Obviously. Not all of us can have 4,200 square feet in Manhattan."

I jostle his shoulder. "And not all of us own the club beneath it either."

"Very true. But it's light? Spacious?"

I nod. "It's probably ridiculous for me to own a place that big just for me, but to be honest, I do get a lot of visitors."

Marco's face takes on a mock horror. "Does this mean you left the Freemans in your home alone? There goes your privacy."

"Please. The concept of privacy went to hell the first night everyone slept over to welcome me to my new place and Phil came out pretending my vibrator was a unicorn horn. This—of course—

was while half the guys were still unpacking boxes." Suddenly I slap my hand to my mouth. "OhmygoddidIsaythat?"

But there's obviously no take backs since Marco's fallen over sideways on the couch. His body's shaking so hard, I have to reach over and snag his plate out of his hand before it ends up on the Turkish rug beneath us. While holding two plates, I pull my knees up and bury my head and begin to moan. "No. Even years later, Phil's causing me hell with that little stunt."

"I am certain Holly got pictures?" Marco manages, demonstrating how close he is with the family.

"Of course. She gave it to me as a nightshirt for Christmas that year," I grumble, which only sets him off again.

"I can only be grateful Holly and her camera were not here one night when I was showing off on the dance floor," Marco shares as he lifts his plate from my hands.

"Oh?" I start to fork up a bite of salad.

He places his hand over mine to still my movement. Oh, this should be good. I turn and tuck my leg beneath me to face him fully. His body starts shaking. "You've have now put together who my brother is? The picture was fairly obvious, yes?"

"Oh yes. I should have put it together based on your resemblance but..." I let out a dreamy sigh, remembering the first time Bristol showed me pictures of her famous husband. "Simon Houde. He's adorable. Bristol's one lucky woman."

Marco coughs. Then coughs again to regain my attention. "Oops. Sorry." I feel the heat rise in my cheeks.

"Remind me to punch my brother later," he says with good humor.

I roll my eyes. "You were saying?"

"Well, I was trying to show off on the dance floor with my sister-in-law—"

"Bristol?" I take a bite of salad.

"No. Evangeline."

I promptly choke, recalling Bristol's confession about her sister being the belle of Broadway. Marco whacks me on the back, and I finally get myself together enough to yell, "I'm fine. I'm okay! Oh, God. I can just picture this. Where was Evangeline's husband?" I remember the bit in the gossip columns about her getting married.

"Montague was watching with Simon and Bristol. We'd attracted quite a crowd."

"I imagine so! Thank goodness you have a no-camera policy."

"And it's for reasons like this." Marco proceeds to tell me how he and Evangeline Brogan were dancing when, "Suddenly I feel this coolness where one should not."

"No," I gasp. "You split your pants?"

"Right there on the dance floor. In front of hundreds. Fortunately, I was wearing all black, so no one noticed, but my darling sister-in-law was laughing at me as she tried to cover..." He thinks for a moment. "*Things* that should not be seen in the event the pants tore more?"

My chest is pressed down to my thighs as I lean forward to place my plate on the table. "What did you do?"

"What could I do? I finished the dance. And then I excused myself and came up here to change." He nods to the elevator that leads down to his private office downstairs.

"What did your family do?" I flop backward, eagerly anticipating the answer.

Instead of answering me, Marco picks up a remote and turns on a song. It's a slow number about not letting go. "How about a bargain?" He puts his dish down, stands, and holds out his hand.

I take it. He pulls me to my feet and brings me around the coffee table so we're not obstructed by furniture. "What's the bargain?" I ask breathlessly as he pulls me into his arms.

"I will answer this and any question you have when the song is over." He pulls me closer to his chest, and I'm momentarily lost in his obsidian eyes.

We sway back and forth with Marco holding one of my hands, the other wrapped around my waist. His eyes never leave my face as the music washes over us. I open my mouth, but no words come out.

Every thought, every question floats away as I'm held in his strong arms, that is until the song starts over. I frown up at him confused. "I thought you said when the song was over?"

His lips are so close, I can practically feel them touch mine when he answers, "I put the song on repeat. Just relax, *mon étoile*. Just dance."

My body melts into his, his hard body absorbing my softness. Every shuffle seems to build an intimate cocoon around us.

And that makes me brave enough to ask him, "What does *mon étoile* mean?"

"My star." Marco's response is whispered against my lips.

I open my mouth to ask why, but his kiss removes my next question from my mind.

16

LYNNE

"So, what's the plan for today," Jenna yawns as she comes into the kitchen. We stayed up late talking about my date with Marco, and I'm left feeling more confused than ever. Fortunately, Dani left to head to Nantucket with Brendan, Em, Jake, Corinna, and Colby as the six of them are flying with everyone's dresses and so Corinna could start the cake. "You realize she," Brendan joked at dinner last night, pointing at Corinna, "is just going to drag me into her kitchen and be mean to me."

Corinna picked up her dessert fork and stabbed it repeatedly into the tiramisu we were devouring at Daniela Trattoria. The entire family burst into laughter except Brendan, who paled. "I give in! I'll help!"

The rest of the Freemans went back to the farm to gather everything they needed. Like me, they had planned on flying out on Monday.

I'm about to answer when the phone rings. "Hold that thought."

"Can I hold a cup of coffee instead?"

"You know where everything is." I pick up the cordless and answer, "Hello?"

"Ms. Bradbury, you have a delivery. Would you like me to bring it up?" my doorman asks.

"Please. Thank you." Wondering if it's a package I forgot I needed for Jenna's wedding, I immediately head to the door after grabbing a tip.

When an enormous bouquet of purple and yellow flowers appears, I rush to help him. "Whoa, Ken. Are those for Jenna?"

"The card has your name on it, Ms. Bradbury."

"Really?" I bury my face in the luscious blooms, forgetting about my doorman. Then regaining myself, I hand him a tip. "Here. I'm so sorry. Thank you for bringing them up."

"Nice to see you have a beau, Ms. Bradbury." He tips an imaginary hat before heading to the elevator.

"Oh, my! Look at those beautiful flowers!" Jenna gushes.

"I thought they might be for you from Finn."

Jenna whacks me before reaching right in and plucking the card out. Slapping it in my hand, she says in a sotto voice, "I bet I know who they're from."

"No way," I scoff. "They're probably from my boss or some..." But my voice trails off when I read the card.

I've barely slept for having you on my mind. Was it the same for you, mon étoile? - MH

My hand holding the card begins to shake. I sit down abruptly as Jenna walks around taking pictures of the flowers from every angle. I read it over and over as she giggles. Belatedly, I realize she's typing. "What are you doing?" I demand.

"Finding out what each flower means from Uncle Phil," Jenna replies cheekily.

I groan. "I'm assuming you didn't get him to sign an NDA first?"

"Well, he's on his way here. I suppose we can get one then."

"Of course he is." I sigh in resignation. "Thank goodness the Lockwood jet can't take in-flight calls or we'd be on FaceTime with Em and Cori."

"That is one perk," Jenna agrees. "God, these flowers are gorgeous, Lynne."

"I know." The words are barely out of my mouth when the pounding starts.

"Open up, little girls," Phil threatens loudly.

"I want to know how come you hate to run," I grumble as I swing my door inward. Phil bursts past me. Ali and Cass hug me before following at a more sedate pace. "But the moment gossip's involved, you manage to sprint city blocks in a matter of minutes."

"And this is why you make the big bucks, Lynne," Ali declares. Cassidy laughs.

Phil sticks his tongue out at both of them before performing his own walk-around. "Pansies, zinnias, morning glories, irises. Flowers say many things. These are telling you that Marco wanted to let you know he finds you thoughtful, that he's going to miss you, there's affection, wisdom, and respect between you both."

Struggling between pleasure and a tiny measure of disappointment there wasn't more meaning, I tease, "And you ran here for that, Phil? You must be so disappointed." Standing, I move into the kitchen. "Now, who wants coffee?"

Ali and Cassidy's hands go up. I'm reaching for the mugs and lining them up on the counter when I hear Phil call my name. "Yes?"

"I didn't mention the last flower."

"Which is?" I lean on the counter.

"There's lilacs in here. Purple lilacs," Phil stresses.

Ali gapes. Cassidy's breath catches. Even Jenna stills. I'm the only one who's lost. "Will one of you explain what that means to people who don't speak native flower?"

Cassidy makes her way over and takes the mug I'm holding out of my hand. Grabbing hold of one of my hands, she murmurs, "Purple lilacs represent the first emotions of love, Lynne. And this isn't a random selection of flowers." Cassidy confirms her guess with her brother, who nods emphatically. "He knew exactly the message he wanted to convey."

"What am I supposed to feel?" My voice is panicked. "What am I supposed to do?"

Jenna comes over to soothe me. "What do you want to do?" She slings her arm around me and hugs me.

Ali and Phil just wait for my response.

I think about schedules and timelines. I consider all the things I was going to do in Nantucket with the family for the next few days and realize I don't have to be on the island for four more days. "If Jenna doesn't mind, I could fly in with Ryan and Jared. That leaves me four days to explore what this might be so I don't go insane."

"What are you going to do up in Nantucket except drive yourself nuts about every last detail which is already perfect? Besides, we can only drink so much." Jenna gives me her blessing.

"I want to give this a shot. I'll regret it if I don't."

"I said something similar about Caleb," Cassidy confides.

My eyes circle the room. "What do I do next? How do I respond to this?"

Phil's blue eyes brighten. "Why don't you ask him to save you a dance at the club tonight?"

Mulling over the idea, I pull out my phone and send Marco a text with just that.

The reply staggers me. *One dance? Non, all the dances.*

I'm not the type of woman to swoon, but this man might make me. "So, is what I wore the other night normal? Because that was a one-of-a-kind dress from Em."

Immediately, we all dash for my closet to find something for me to wear to Redemption.

Before we reach my bedroom, I grab Jenna. "Are you sure? This is your wedding week…"

"And if you think I don't want the sister of my heart happy, you're crazy. Seriously, you're actually doing me and Finn a favor. With you out of the guest apartment, Finn and I can enjoy a few uninhibited pre-wedding festivities."

Phil yells, "Stop. You're sharing that apartment with me and Jason as well."

Jenna shouts back. "Like you haven't done it all before."

"Okay. I get the point. It's a good thing I'm staying out of the love shack as long as possible," I tease.

Jenna grabs my cheeks. "Enjoy whatever it is you find with Marco, Lynne. Don't hold back. Just be you."

Prying her hands away, I smile so wide my dimple pops. "I promise. No holding back."

"Good. Now, let's go rescue your closet."

And together we head into my bedroom to find exactly what to wear when one needs something more than Redemption.

They need freedom.

17

LYNNE

Black leather pants and spiked thin-heeled boots. A bright blue shell that according to Cassidy, "Does amazing things to your eyes." And a beaded knit shawl to top it that barely skims the top of my hips. Ali declared I looked like a million dollars. Phil said I resembled a present to unwrap. Jenna announced I looked sexy and comfortable.

I just hope I didn't make a fool of myself as the car pulls up to the main entrance to Redemption where a line wraps around the perimeter of the building. "You'd better not have cursed me with your split-pants story, Marco," I vow.

"Excuse me, ma'am?" my driver asks.

"Nothing. I'm sorry."

"Not a problem. We're here. Let me come around."

I patiently wait for the driver's assistance. When I emerge from the car, I follow the instructions from Marco and walk past the line. I can practically feel the hissing from the females in line as I stride confidently straight up to Louie. "Long time no see," I greet him.

He unfolds himself from behind the podium and engulfs me in a warm hug. "Hold on just a second." Pulling a phone from his hip, he types something quickly. "Marco's on his way. Now, before he gets here, tell me how you did it." Louie's eyes are as bright as his gold tooth.

"Did what?" I ask, confused.

"How you... Hey, Marco." Louie grins over my shoulder.

I feel his arm slide around my waist. "*Mon étoile*, I'm sorry to make you wait." He brushes a kiss to my temple.

"That's all right. I just got here." I smile my reassurance up at him.

"Jesus, Marco, you didn't give me a chance to grill her," Louie complains good-naturedly.

"Or torment her like you did Colby the first night you met him?" Both men laugh. I mentally remind myself to ask someone about that later. But Marco continues. "Then I arrived just in time. Eleven?"

"Everything will be ready," Louie assures him.

Marco nods and begins to guide me. I wave over my shoulder.

Louie's smile softens, and he sends me a wink just as I disappear behind the velvet curtain into Marco's world for another night. Only this time, it's so very different as I'm led right to the dance floor and into his arms.

Hours later, I'm downing a bottle of water at one of the high-top tables when Marco asks, "Did you eat before you came?"

"Depends on your definition of eating. We munched on some cheese and crackers while I put my outfit together and said goodbye." I lean forward so I can be heard over P!nk.

"That's an *aperitif*."

"It was consumable."

"Come with me," he urges.

I hold up my water and wave it in question. He plucks it from my hand and leaves it on the table. Weaving us around until we reach a private door, Marco reaches for a black key card to unlock it. Behind it is an elevator. Once we're inside, the music is immediately muffled. "Is this the one to your office?" I ask curiously.

"It is. And I have a surprise there for us."

"I assume it involves putting something in my mouth?" As Marco begins to laugh, I blurt out, "Oh my God, did that just come out?"

"Oh, the comments I could make, lovely Lynne."

I punch his hard abs before I trail my fingers over his stomach. "When do you find the time to work out?" My voice is distracted.

His breathing is jagged. "When I can. Your touch distracts me."

That doesn't stop me from running my fingers up his muscled stomach to his chest. When my fingers find the open space where his shirt is unbuttoned, we're both breathing as hard as if we were still dancing. It's Marco who breaks the spell we're under. "Come. Let's get some refreshments before we indulge in dessert." He takes my hand away from his body and pulls me over to a long black sofa where a table is set with white candles and several silver-domed dishes.

I settle on the couch while Marco quickly lifts the cloche and explains the selection of finger foods. "There's quite a selection," I remark offhandedly.

"I wasn't sure what you'd like." Marco leans forward to spread some olive tapenade on a toast point before holding it to my lips. Yuck.

"I'm surprised you didn't just look up the menu from the other night." I lean around him and spear myself a barbecue meatball on a tiny fork. "We devoured the hell out of these."

Marco's face blanks before he puts down the toast without taking a bite himself. "I didn't think of that."

"Just ordered a standard selection of items for whichever woman you choose to bring to your office?" I throw out. Ignoring the sting of irritation when he doesn't contradict my words, I toss the fork on the tiny plate. "See the difference is, I was more impressed with the you I met yesterday."

I'm about to stand when Marco grips my wrist. Expecting him to bring it to his wrist, I'm surprised when he wraps it around the back of his neck. My heart thumps inside my chest when it's my other hand he kisses. "I'm the same man you met the other night, Lynne." He shifts so we're so close to each other I can practically count his eyelashes.

"Are you?" I murmur as his lips touch my brow.

I feel like yesterday I gained some part of Marco Houde not many people have experienced—the man in the light. Tonight, he's the epitome of the dark, from his custom-made suit to the expression on his face. And like every other fool before me, I'm sucked into it despite the chill that races up my spine.

I'm afraid if I go down the dark path, I may never see the light again. But as Marco whispers a kiss across my lips, I let myself weaken.

I whimper when his lips settle on mine more firmly. Taking the lead, Marco leads me on a sensual dance that begins with a flirtation. His teeth nip at my full lower one. But when I try to reciprocate, he retreats with a diabolical laugh.

Excitement begins to pulsate in my veins as he slides his hand up, raising my shawl over my head. I duck my head long enough for him to dispose of the garment. His hands cup my heavy breasts, rubbing the nipples back and forth as he ruthlessly plunders my lips.

Slowly, I find myself being lowered backward until Marco's lying atop of me. I tear my mouth away to get some breath, and my eyes land on the silver domes. Warning bells sound in my head as his hand smooths over my rear. "Yes. I will have you, Lynne." Marco bites my nipple through my shirt just as a speaker sounds.

"Boss? Just checking to see if you've headed to your place yet." It's a cheerful voice, but their intrusion into the dark reality Marco's cultivated is like a bucket of ice water over us both.

We both still, before Marco bites off a French curse. He slides off me to go punch a button while I take stock of everything that's happened.

It was a setup. I was supposed to be a hookup.

Well, aren't Marco's plans about to change?

18

MARCO

I'm stunned when Lynne saunters into the elevator with her shawl tossed over her shoulder like nothing's just happened between us. Without thinking, I slam my hand in the way of the closing doors. "You're lying," I accuse her. "You want me."

She negligently shrugs her shoulder as if the red-hot burning passion between us is something she can feel with any man any day. "I never denied that. What I said is I refuse to be treated like any other woman. How many have you brought up here for a quick dinner and a tumble on your sofa?"

Unconsciously, my head twists around to eye the setup I instructed my head bartender to lay out earlier. And I cringe remembering his comment: "Been a while for you. Good to see you back in the game."

And while I gave him a glare that should have peeled the skin from his body, I can't deny Lynne's question. My silence is my answer.

Leaning against the back wall, she declares, "I am worth so much more than trite moves you've used on other women."

Irritated she picked up on them in the first place, because she's right, I bite out, "Well, there's plenty of them around," though I can't imagine a single one.

I only want her. This one frustrating, smart, enchanting female who refuses to let me take the easy way out because I can.

Hurt flashes across her face for a second before a cool mask drops down. "Well, aren't you lucky you can walk straight into hell via your own private elevator to pick one? Now, if you'll excuse me, I'd like to leave."

Startled by her words, I take an inadvertent step back as I say, "No, wait. Lynne, I'm sor—"

But the closing of the elevator doors in my face reduces my apology to nothing.

"*Trou du cul.*" I call myself a jackass before I slip my phone from my pocket. I try to call Louie to stop her, but either he can't or won't pick up.

Fuck, I'll never make it in time.

Frantically, I push the call button. "Come on." I pound my hand against the door in frustration, still holding my phone, which chooses that moment to ring. The elevator doors open and close as I answer.

Before I can say a word, Louie announces, "She's gone. Slipped into the car she hired and hightailed it out of here." Before I can make a sound, he disconnects the call.

I whirl around and hurl my phone ineffectually against the couch. My fingertips brush against one another as I recall the way Lynne's smooth skin felt against them when I peeled her shawl over her head. The way her eyes became hooded as I smoothed my hand over her breast. The way her body arched into mine...

And the way she shoved me away when we heard the voice over the speaker.

"Foolish idiot," I curse myself again. "What are you thinking to even touch her? She is worth ten—no, a thousand—of you. Just forget about her."

Reaching for one of the glasses of wine on the table, I tip it to my lips when I taste her. Jerking back, I find my lips have pressed to the same spot on the glass where hers rested. "Do I feel like this because I hurt her or because I care for her?" I wonder aloud.

"I suspect it's both." I'm startled when I hear my brother's voice.

"I didn't hear you come up." A vast understatement. I gesture my brother to sit down across from me.

After lowering himself into the chair, he observes, "You were out of it. Louie said I'd find you up here. What happened?"

I open my mouth to tell him, but I'm afraid if I do, I'm going to tell him all of it—back to when he left for school in England. "An apology I need to make."

Simon thinks about my words. "For the longest time, I wanted to be like you."

I was in the process of swallowing some Bordeaux accented by Lynne, so I promptly choke. "Good God, why? Look at everything you have—who you've become."

Simon draws in a breath. "Because you're the kind of man who always seems to know what to do in every situation. You have such ease about you."

"Me?" I'm incredulous.

A bark of laughter escapes Simon. "The first night I met Bristol, I tried to act just like my big brother."

I'm still lost. "Why would you be anything but yourself with a woman you care about?"

"I think that was Evangeline's point when she began our onstage halitosis war. She wanted her sister to see me for the man I am. Whoever the woman is—"

"Lynne Bradbury," I blurt out, feeling uncomfortably like a boy out of the schoolroom with a crush instead of a man with a much more salacious interest.

A silence descends between us when suddenly Simon throws his head back and roars with laughter. "Brother, are you certain you want to take that woman on?"

"What do you mean?" I demand. "Lynne is lovely, compassionate..."

"And has a mind as sharp as Bristol's."

I can't refute that, so I just tip my head in acknowledgement.

Simon, being no slouch in the intellectual department himself, puts one and one together to understand my mood quickly. "Let me take a stab in the dark. Instead of learning her as an individual woman, you laid out your patented 'let's go to bed' scene." With a tsk, he reaches over and plucks a plump strawberry from the pile. Biting into it, he mumbles, "Needs some updating."

"And what would you suggest? What did you use to get Bristol in bed?" Not that I really want to know, but he's pushed me so far the words just fly from my mouth.

Simon grins, and there's no trace of the Tony-award-winning Broadway actor across from me. There's only my brother—the brother I have and for whom I would do unspeakable things to ensure his happiness. While I'm still staggering under the weight of the love I feel for him, he hits me with something unexpected. "Cilantro."

"What does that garbage food topping have to do with..."

"I ate a bunch of it to put Evangeline off our onstage kiss. We were fighting afterwards when Bristol came up and kissed me," he remembers fondly.

"How does that—" I start to ask impatiently.

Simon stands. I do the same. "You're an enigma, Marco, and I'm your brother. I've loved you my whole life and always will. But you want this woman to share herself with you without getting to know you? Think about it. Would you do the same?"

No. The answer comes to my mind swiftly. But how do I let her in without destroying the carefully constructed walls I built to keep my past at bay?

Simon's chuckle brings me back. "And I can see I lost your attention. I'll head out for now." He starts to head to the elevator, his training in theater arts making his moments so fluid it's like he's gliding across the floor. Just before he reaches the door, I call out, "Was there something you needed?"

Simon shakes his head. "Bristol and Evangeline were driving me insane. Monty's in class, so I couldn't tell him to come drag his wife away."

I chuckle, something I never expected to be able to do amid my own mess. But Simon's next words clear my thoughts of everything but certainty that everything I did was righteous though no one would see it that way.

"Really, Marco, I just wanted to be with the one man in the world who I always knew I could count on. I just wanted to tell you, *je t'aime toujours, mon frère*."

"I always love you too, brother," I manage hoarsely. Surging to my feet, I wrap Simon in a huge hug.

While he has me close, my brother takes a moment to scold me. "Let her see the real you, Marco. Not all this." He waves his hand. "This is just a wrapper around the greatest man I've ever known."

As Simon slips away, I stride back over to the couch to grab my cell before leaving the mess behind me.

Simon's right. I need to think about Lynne where the real me spent time with her.

And that's not here.

Texting Louie that I'm done for the night, I head upstairs to figure out how to correct this monumental disaster of an evening that was completely my fault.

I press my hand against my stomach as a hollow ache begins. I also need to plan how to make myself vulnerable to a woman. And willingly embracing the idea is terrifying.

19

LYNNE

My house line rings, notifying me the doorman's calling. "Good morning, Ken," I answer with a sleepy yawn. A quick glance at my clock shows me it's only ten. Considering I fell into my own bed around four after spending hours with Marco's lips on me in his office, I'm feeling lazy.

"Good morning, Ms. Bradbury. A Mr. Marco Houde is here to see you. Are you accepting visitors?"

Before my doorman can finish saying Marco's first name, I'm leaping from the bed to grab my robe. Dashing to the bathroom, I rip open a package of wipes. *Thank God I took off my makeup last night* is prevalent in my mind. Secondary is that with a quick flip of my brush, my bob looks relatively decent. I'm about to shove my toothbrush in my mouth when I answer, "Yes."

"Then I'll send him right up."

Not waiting another second longer, I shove the mint-flavored paste in my mouth. Hoping my teeth forgive me for neglect, I rinse, spit, and wipe the residue off just as I hear the knock on my door. I make a mad dash for the door. After a calming breath, I fling it open.

And my thighs clench together. God, how is it possible for one man to be so damn sexy?

Sporting aviator shades, a white tee that molds his broad shoulders and flat stomach, and worn jeans, my body is cursing me for being a fool twenty times over for not taking up his invitation and staying last night. "Marco. This is a surprise." I chastise myself mentally for not thinking of something more intriguing to say.

"Good morning, Lynne. May I come in?" He slides off his glasses, and the evidence of a sleepless night is noticeable on his face.

Stepping back, I let him into the foyer which leads right into the kitchen and family room. "Would you like some coffee?"

"If it's not too much trouble."

"I was going to make some for myself," I tell him. It's not a falsehood. It would have been true in a few more hours. "Make yourself comfortable."

Quickly, I pull down a few mugs. As I wait for my magical Keurig to do its business, I call out, "Do you need cream?" and jump when his hands land on my shoulders.

"No, black is fine."

"Christ, you startled me," I gasp. "Wear a damn bell."

There's an unmistakable tension between us that has nothing to do with desire and everything to do with uncertainty. Fortunately, the beeping of the coffee maker intercedes at that moment. I hand him his coffee. "Why don't you take a seat at the bar?"

"Will you join me?"

I frown. "Why wouldn't I?"

"Perhaps because I acted like a spoiled child last night."

I slide to the side and pull the cream out of the fridge. After pouring some into my freshly brewed cup, I take a welcome sip. "Not used to a woman declining an offer of a night in your bed?"

"I don't make them that often. So, no. I'm not," Marco says flatly.

I promptly choke on my coffee. "You expect me to believe that? What happened to no lies between us?"

Placing his mug down, Marco approaches me warily. "That's why I'm here. I owe you an apology for implying all I wanted was a night of sex."

"Then what do you want?" I challenge him. Before he can speak, I plow on. "And don't try to tell me you can't get laid by one of the many women at Redemption."

"If I wanted relief, I have a hand, *mon étoile*. And trust me, I've made use of it before."

Comments like that are just cruel. I envision myself throwing my coffee on his pristine clothing so he'll be forced whip them off, showing me the remarkable body I know lies beneath. Cursing myself as much as I want to curse Marco, I set aside my own drink before I turn that little fantasy into a reality. Even though the one I really want to see is where he has his hand wrapped around his own cock, stroking...

Tuning back in, I find Marco watching me intently. "I want what we started the other day at my home. I crave the woman who opened up to me, who made me smile and laugh. She's captivated me unlike anyone I've met in far too long. And like a fool, I rushed things."

"That's a lot to take in," I admit honestly.

"Why? We promised no lies." Marco steps closer so just the tips of our fingers touch on my marble countertop.

"Because of who I am, how I was raised. That's not how I see myself."

Carefully, he lifts my hand. Bringing it to his lips, he kisses the inside of my wrist. "Can I spend the day with you? Just be with you? I want to experience whatever it is you do in the light."

Light, dark. Maybe I was right the day we rode up to his place for lunch. There are two sides to this complicated man, and he seems to understand that both live inside him.

The question is why?

"All right." I hold up my free hand as a smile breaks out across his face. "But be forewarned, I'm running errands all day for the wedding that I had planned on doing in Nantucket. Now I'm going to be scrambling for what I need here."

Marco's chest rises and falls. "I haven't said thank you for that either." His tone is laced with both pleasure and sorrow.

Light and dark. The sides of Marco Houde few see.

"For what?"

"For staying to explore this." He pulls me against him. But where I expect him to kiss me, he just holds me in an embrace so sweet, I think my body begins to melt in his arms.

After a while, he pulls back. "But, I think New York should not see you like this, *non*? You should find clothes, *mon étoile*."

I back away and head in the direction of my bedroom. "Make yourself at home." Without waiting for a reply, I dash away to put on something to wear to grab some sexy gifts for Jenna.

And maybe for myself too.

I'M grateful the exclusive lingerie salon that's tucked away a few floors above Madison Avenue was able to fit me in. I would have found something on the island at one of the boutiques, but Jenna won't be expecting this.

What I love about Pour Vous is each piece is one of a kind. No two sizes have the same style whether it's a brassiere and panty set or a negligée like I'm holding up in a rich chocolate silk with cream-colored lace. It might cost me a small fortune, but my best friend is getting married.

Instead of being uncomfortable, Marco is intrigued. He's neither hovering behind me nor disengaged, both of which I predicted would have occurred. No, he's meandering around the store, paying special attention to some of the silk robes and maternity wear.

After I've handed my selection to the sales associate, I approach him. His large fingers are delicately touching a sky-blue maternity robe. "For Bristol?" I ask, knowing Bristol is pregnant with her second child.

"I would purchase it for my brother to surprise her with, but I don't know what size is appropriate."

"Let's find out." I get the attention of the associate I was working with. After a few quick questions, she checks her tablet.

"A medium would be best. Fortunately, that's what the blue comes in." Discreetly, she slips away.

"What did you ask her?" Marco asks as he lifts the robe off the hook.

"I just gave her Bristol's general size. For something else, I would need more specifics."

"Gotcha." His eyes scan the silks and lace dotting the store before he asks, "Did you get what you came in for?"

I give an emphatic nod. "I did."

Marco shifts slightly, not an overt motion, but one that makes me very aware of his masculinity. "And what about for you, Lynne? Did you select a little scrap of nothing for yourself designed to drive a man wild thinking of you wearing it?"

I shake my head no.

"Why not?"

I lean forward to answer, "Because when I slide on scraps of lace, I choose them for me first. Always. Shouldn't I want to make myself feel sexy first?"

His breathing accelerates as I step back. "I'm going to pay for my purchases."

As I start to walk away, Marco stops me by calling my name. "Yes?"

"Do some of those purchases include items for yourself?"

My lips purse. A few seconds of heated silence pass between us before I answer, "I couldn't resist."

I hear him mutter, "*Merde*," before I take my first step.

A proud feminine smile curves my lips. *Oh, Marco. If only you hadn't been such a presumptuous ass last night, you might have seen the strapless bra and thong I was wearing.*

I glance back at him while my packages are being wrapped. Judging by the heat in his gaze, he's come to the same conclusion.

Regrets, Marco. You never know when they'll come back to haunt you. Me? I don't regret leaving last night. I'm proud of myself. I may not be everyone's ideal woman, but I have my full measure of pride.

Even if I struggled to find it.

20

MARCO

"I suppose I should go?" I ask uncertainly after we get back to Lynne's after a day spent together.

"Are you in such a hurry?" She kicks off her shoes in the hallway.

"Not at all. I didn't want to presume."

Shoving a package containing wine in my direction, she orders, "Make yourself useful, Marco. Opener is in the drawer next to the dishwasher. I need to put these in my closet."

"You're asking me to stay?" I need her to confirm somehow I'm being absolved for my poor behavior the night before.

With a mischievous glance, Lynne closes the distance between us, her arms still laden with bags of this and that. "Either you're abjectly sorry, or you're doing your damnedest to end up in my bed."

"Both, if I'm being honest." Then I internally cringe.

Humor makes her face beautiful in the setting light of the city streaming through her windows. I want to lean down and capture her lips beneath mine. "Well, that's more honest than last night."

I wince. "Ouch. I deserved that."

Lynne laughs and my soul soars at the sound. "Open the wine, and then I'll show you the wonders of an Instant Pot." She pads on bare feet down the hall.

I'm grinning goofily before I process her words. "*Mon étoile*, what is an Instant Pot?"

"You'll see," she calls over her shoulder as she disappears inside a room.

Turning into her kitchen, I open the drawer and find the corkscrew. I quickly open the wine and leave it to breathe just as Lynne saunters into the kitchen.

"Now, tell the truth?"

"I promised you already. With you, always."

Lynne goes into her refrigerator and pulls out several bricks of cheese including, I'm pleased to note, gruyère. "Tell me how you feel about gorging on outrageously decadent mac 'n' cheese."

"It sounds amazing. But it won't be ready for us to eat soon enough."

Lynne just shakes her head. "Oh, ye of little faith." She turns around and hefts a device that resembles a small robot off the counter behind her. "It will be done in ten minutes if we worship Susie-Q appropriately."

I spin around thinking there's someone else in the room with us, but Lynne's staring adoringly at the inanimate object. "That thing can make edible food in ten minutes it takes chefs hours to put together brilliantly?"

Lynne wraps her arms around the wide base. Her voice turns fierce. "Don't worry, Susie. We've won this battle over and over. What's one more cynic?"

Enchanted by another facet to the delightful Lynne Bradbury, I try to school my face long enough to ask, "What can I do to help?"

"Pour the wine." Lynne lets go of the machinery long enough long to collect noodles, mustard powder, paprika, and some measuring instruments.

"Glasses?" I ask, moving back toward the wine.

"Cabinet above where you are." Lynne returns her attention to our dinner.

As I pour, I wince at the sound of raw noodles being poured into the pot. I wonder if I can talk Lynne into takeout if I add more to her glass. "Aren't you supposed to cook them first?" I ask tentatively.

"Marco, trust me." Lynne's voice is full of exasperation.

Deciding I'll need more wine than Lynne, I take a drink before I return to the island. Placing both glasses in easy reach, I bravely ask, "What do you need me to do?"

Beaming, Lynne finishes adding the spices and attaches the lid before sliding a box shredder across the island. "Let me prepare the salad if you don't mind shredding cheese."

"I'm happy to help however I can."

Her smile makes me satisfied with salad being a perfectly acceptable dinner

~

"I'VE GOT TO STOP EATING," I moan as I plow through my second helping that Lynne and her miracle appliance Susie-Q produced. "It is fabulous."

Around a bite of food, Lynne's laughing at me. "Told you so."

"In the same amount of time it takes to microwave a meal, you made a culinary delight."

Swallowing, she corrects me. "No, I made some good old-fashioned deliciousness."

"That's for sure. You know I would have taken you out."

"I eat out constantly when I travel. I enjoy spending time outside of a restaurant with people just talking."

I reach for the bottle of wine and top off her glass and my own before bringing up what happened. "And last night?"

Lynne flushes. "I was a brat, and I owe you an apology for that."

"It's the other way around. You were right." This woman is so special, she deserves more than the tired and trite.

She frowns before leaning forward to exchange her food for her glass. "I hide my true feelings behind a mask when I feel uncomfortable."

"Was it because I brought you to my office?" I'm ready to kick my own ass.

"No, that wasn't it." I become tense when her brows lower thoughtfully. "It was the expectation, the assumption, we were going to happen. Like I was supposed to fall in line because you'd decided I was supposed to."

I open my mouth to argue, but what comes out is, "God, that is what it looked like, *n'est-ce pas?*"

Lynne pats my hand. I quickly capture her fingers and lift her wrist up and kiss the inside.

"Why do you do that?" she whispers breathlessly.

"This?" I brush my lips against her skin again. "I never had the desire to before you. It's as if I can get closer to all your senses by touching you here."

"What do you mean?" Her voice is raspy.

I pull the wine from her hand and place our glasses on the table. Taking both her hands, I face her. "Despite whatever crosses your lips, I hear what your heart's saying." I lift her left wrist and press my lips against it.

"I can hear the beat of your heart as blood rushes through it. The skin is so delicate, it's almost fragile, even if the woman inside is stronger than anyone I've ever met." Her right wrist is given the same treatment.

"You carry the scent you wear here. It's mixed with the most intoxicating taste."

"What's that?"

"You."

She rises to her knees, putting her just slightly above eye level. "Marco?"

"*Oui?*" I want her so badly after my hands innocuously brushed against hers, my cock might explode.

"This is how you should have tried to seduce me last night." Then Lynne sinks her fingers into my hair before taking the initiative to kiss me for the first time.

21

LYNNE

My fingers fall through his hair until they find purchase on his broad shoulders. I don't deepen the kiss with the passion we exchanged last night, but with a well of tenderness that's built up as we've laughed all day. Marco's kept me off-balance with forthrightness and with humor. It's disarmed me in a way I didn't expect.

Then again, I didn't expect him.

His eyes remain open as our lips touch gently over and over. My breath hitches in my throat as his hands grip my hips tightly, the pads of his fingers pressing in so tightly I wonder if there will be bruises.

He wants me, and knowing that increases my own desire.

I push myself off the couch and hold out my hand. "Be with me?"

He places a bare foot on the floor before taking my outstretched hand. "What will happen between us will be so much more than that, *mon étoile.*"

A shiver of anticipation courses through my body as I lead him down the hall and into my bedroom.

～

IT MAY BE minutes or hours later, but my skin's burning everywhere Marco touches it.

I feel like I'm being branded as he uses his hands, his lips, his fingers to caress every inch of my skin as he peels me out of my clothes. Any doubts I had about giving myself to this man are erased as his hot breath rakes over my skin, raising every single hair on my body as he murmurs, *"C'est très bon."*

It's magnificent because it's him. But I can't get the words out because his mouth closes over one of my nipples—nipping and sucking, turning the tips so sensitive that when the cool air touches them, I moan in sweet agony.

My legs part in agony and in anticipation. "I want you," I gasp.

"No more than I want you."

"Lie," I challenge breathlessly.

But he doesn't respond. That moment is when he decides to slide off the bed before shucking off his jeans and briefs. And if I thought I was close to coming while he was touching me, it has nothing on when he reaches down and grabs the base of his cock and begins to drag his fingers up toward the head. Then he does it again as I shove myself to a kneeling position.

"I want to be the one to do that." Only I want so much more. I want to cover the head with my mouth, to slide my tongue over the bubble of precum that's beginning to form. I want to lick up the taste of him as I stroke him and make him wild. My tongue wets my lower lip in anticipation.

He stops and plants his feet like a long-ago warrior. "Do you really?"

Dragging my eyes upward, I find his chin tucked downward. "Oh yeah."

Marco leans down. "Well, so do I." He reaches around behind me before tucking his fingers into the notch between my legs. "So wet." His voice is a seductive purr as he eases in a finger, then two.

My back bows even as my core clenches down on him. "Not fair," I pant as I reach for him.

Before I can grab onto him, Marco tumbles me onto my back. He straddles my head before bowing his own down. "Like this. But just for a while," he warns.

I nod, just before I bury my nose into the scent of him. "Hmm, okay." I swipe my tongue up along his shaft, coating it with moisture, before letting out a long sigh. Dreamily, I realize I want to bottle his taste for my own personal pleasure. I cup one of his balls in my hand to massage it as I flick my tongue directly beneath the head of his cock when suddenly, I grab onto his ass with all my might.

Marco's mouth has joined his fingers in his ministrations. "You should be rewarded for that mouth, Lynne."

"What you're doing is...ooh!" My hips roll as the flicks of his tongue pantomime the kisses we shared. Marco grips my hips to hold them still before placing his whole mouth over me.

Then his fingers are replaced with his tongue spearing inside me, and I'm chanting his name over and over as he hurls me over the edge between sanity and ecstasy.

The sensations that tear through my soul are unlike anything I've ever experienced before. Any orgasm I've experienced in the past is almost insipid in comparison to this. I somehow manage to slide my hand up the inside of Marco's thigh as he gentles me. There's a spot where the hair on his legs meets the smooth skin of his ass. My fingers are trailing along it when I feel myself being spun around on the bed.

Black eyes sear me. As if I were a rag doll, Marco drapes me across my bed before reaching down and pulling out a condom from his wallet. Quickly sliding on protection, he smooths a hand up my thigh before catching it in the crook of his elbow. "It will be deeper this way," he promises.

"Oh, my." I'm not even aware of the fact I've said the words aloud as Marco begins to press forward. Then he surges forward until he can nuzzle my ear, whispering words of encouragement to cause me to relax as his long shaft presses in. Marco continues to stretch me until I feel the heavy weight of his sac against my buttocks.

Then, he slowly withdraws.

I clutch at him with the one hand he's not trapped with his body.

"Shh, *mon étoile*. Slow and easy." He pushes forward again.

"You're going to cause me to die."

His chuckle reverberates against me as he begins the torture all over again.

My internal muscles clamp down on him as I fight to breathe, to find the way back to sanity. "Marco, please." I push up as he thrusts down.

"That's it. That's right," he groans as the flutters become stronger.

I shake my head back and forth on the pillow. No, it's not possible his cock just grew inside me. A mixture of disbelief and desire causes me to tremble within the cage of his arms.

"More. Take it all. Take all of me." He's thrusting without control now.

Knowing I can, I push back as hard as I can. Marco bends his head and sucks on the top of my breast, my nipple, nipping at my ear, before capturing my mouth in a kiss so searing it causes my eyes to cross.

And my pussy to clamp down on him tightly before exploding in ripples all around.

He thrusts hard against me before he roars his release.

My heart pounding, I curl up without any thought in my mind. I only recognize the warmth of his arms as he cradles me close. Knowing I'm not alone, I drift off.

22

MARCO

After sex, I've always felt a need to escape almost as soon as the act itself was complete.

But not this time—not with this woman.

I'm not really sure how to feel about it. There's something about the way her fingers grip my sides, how her breath rustles against the hair on my chest, soothes instead of terrifies me.

And she has no idea because her lashes are fanned out across her cheeks as she's asleep.

Cautiously, I ease to her side and slide out of her, missing the tight heat of her body immediately. I'll stay just for a few moments. Just long enough to make sure she'll come to no harm. Reaching behind me for a tissue on the nightstand, I discard of the condom with ease. Lynne has tucked her hands beneath her cheek, lips parted in sleep. Little puffs of air cause my eyelashes to flutter.

"*Mon étoile*, now I know why the nobles used to worship the stars." Cautiously, I brush back a strand of hair that's stuck to her cheek. "It's because they knew they could live off starlight forever once they found it."

Her brows scrunch adorably before smoothing. She twists a bit and frowns before dragging her bare legs up to her chest. Realizing she must be chilled, I work the blanket out from beneath us. Immediately, Lynne snuggles deep, secure and content.

Everything someone should feel after they've had the kind of sexual experience we just did. Only one of us can't.

Because I didn't deserve to take her to begin with.

I begin to count backward from one hundred. When I reach seventy-six, I debate whether she's asleep enough to slide from the bed.

That's when I feel my heart crack.

Lynne's head has rolled slightly, and she's pressed her lips to the inside of my wrist. "I understand." Azure eyes connect with mine, and for a terrifying moment, I think she means the secrets I'm tired of carrying. I open my mouth to explain when she guts me by whispering a single word. "Stay?"

Stay. I was never asked to stay by... I quickly slam the door closed on those thoughts. I roll into the alluring woman next to me until she's on her back. Looking down into her shadowed eyes, I murmur, "If I stay, I doubt you'll sleep much."

She pretends to contemplate my threat, but I don't let her think for too long. If I do, she might recognize the error of her ways in the shadows surrounding me—the shadows I'm so used to living in.

And this woman? Well, she makes me want to stay not just the night but in the light.

And I can't.

I lost my honor too many years ago to be able to do that.

23

LYNNE

I convinced Marco to stay while I packed today since I leave tomorrow morning for Nantucket. "This way, you choose what you want to do with me all night," I called as I ran past him with the packages I'd stored in my guest room.

The lascivious smile he sent my way told me he definitely had plans. Boy, am I glad I picked up a few pieces of new lingerie at the boutique.

Barefoot, shirtless, and wearing only the jeans he had on yesterday, Marco quietly observes while I drag one already packed suitcase close to the door. Meanwhile, I fill a second with my clothes. Then I quickly arrange the contents for an enormous carry-on and my laptop bag on the counter. "How long did you say you're going for?"

I blow a piece of hair out my face. "The weekend."

He bursts into laughter. "Are you afraid the island is going to be ambushed and you will need to sell your clothing to raise money to return to Manhattan?"

"Cute."

He gives a negligent shrug as if he's been told that many times before. I'm sure he has. Ignoring the sting that causes, I haughtily inform him, "One of those suitcases is for Jenna's honeymoon."

Clarity replaces humor. "Ahh. There are things she didn't want her intended to see?"

"Exactly. And as maid of honor, one of my jobs is to help her."

"You mean to reduce her husband to a puddle of mush early on in the marriage."

Narrowing my eyes, I cock out a hip. "Have you been married before?"

"No, but I have seen my sisters-in-law do this to their husbands." He's thoughtful for a moment. "I always thought it was because they are biological sisters, their machinations are more diabolical than most."

"It's not; it's because we're women, and we'll do anything to help a sister out," I drawl.

His face pales slightly. I immediately become concerned. "What? What is it?"

"I just had a terrifying thought of Bristol and Evangeline meeting the Freemans. For a moment, I became alarmed."

"Oh, that?" I wave a hand. "It's already happened. Nothing to worry about."

"And the earth is still spinning?"

"World's still going round, Marco," I joke. I walk around searching for my printed schedule of wedding events. "Now, where did I put that folder?"

"What does it look like? I can help you look," he offers.

"Aqua blue. Lots of notes written on the cover." Marco smirks before sliding to the side slightly. When he shifts, it magically appears next to him on the counter. "There it is."

"What's in there?"

"Wedding plans."

"I'm surprised they're not on your computer." He nods at my Mac.

"They are. This is in the event there's a power issue. Cassidy always sends everything in triplicate." At the confused look on his face, I explain, "Phone, computer, and print. She's the most organized and anal-retentive person I know. As I consider myself one of those people, that says a lot."

He smiles, and I'm transfixed by the slash of white through his darkly Mediterranean features. "God, you're breathtaking."

Capturing me around the waist, Marco kisses my lips softly before whispering, "If you knew what was beneath the surface, I wonder if you would say the same thing."

I shiver under his unwavering stare. "Will you tell me?"

He doesn't hesitate before answering, "No."

Frustrated, I turn away, grabbing the folder so I can pack it. After jamming it in with all of the other things I need, I zip that bag. "Okay. I think I'm all set other than cosmetics." I turn on my heel to make my way to my bedroom.

"Lynne." His voice stops me in place.

I turn slightly.

"Maybe in time. I never have shared this part of myself with another soul." He stuns me with his complete openness. "Not my family, nor Cori. I mean no one."

Turning completely to face him, I give him the same. "My parents hated me because I wasn't perfect. They thought I was repugnant and repulsive."

"That's a lie," he says flatly.

Offended, I turn away. "No, it's not."

"No, not what you said. The lie is that you are none of those things. They should have been proud of their daughter and prouder of the woman you've become. They are those awful words because they do not accept the beautiful woman you are."

I reach out to place my hand against the wall for support as the force of his words almost drive me to my knees.

Behind me, I hear the slap of his feet as he approaches. "Will you tell me?" His words echo my own.

My head falls back against his bare chest when his warmth envelops me. He molds his chest to my back. His arms encircle my stomach, smoothing over the naturally convex bump. His hands cross at the wrist, fingers digging into my slightly dimpled thighs. All the imperfections people who were supposed to love me punished me for having, Marco cherished last night with his mouth and body. "What do you want to know?" I ask raggedly.

"Everything." But I'm astonished when he steps back and spins me in his arms to embrace me hard. "But there is a time and a place for it. And the day before you leave for a wedding is neither, *non*? We have time."

Grateful for the reprieve, I nuzzle against his chest. "I'm almost done. What do you want to do today?" I pull back so I can see his answer.

His smile is almost boyish with good humor. "You are not the only one with errands, *mon étoile*. Why don't I leave for a few to change? You do the same, and then we will spend the rest of the day together?"

"And the night?" I rush to add in. If I'm going to be away for the next four days, I want to get my fill of Marco before I board the plane. But then an idea pops into my head.

Maybe I don't have to miss him. Hmm, it's something to think about.

He draws a finger down my nose before pressing a kiss to the tip of it. "Yes."

"Then it sounds perfect." Just like the man in front of me.

"Two hours," he decrees before sauntering in the direction of my bedroom where he left his loafers and shirt.

God don't let this be a crazy dream where I wake up alone in a city by myself, I plead silently after he leaves and I lock the doors. After all, what does a man as perfect as him want with someone with as many issues as a woman like me?

Unable to bear the ghosts of my past trying to answer the question for me, I head in the direction of my shower.

24

MARCO

Lynne falls out of the elevator laughing. Dropping a shopping bag of food on the counter, she proclaims, "Did you see the look on Bristol's face when you walked in with your arm around me?"

I snicker. "I bet you my darling sister-in-law thinks she set us up. Little does she know..."

Lynne twirls perfectly until she's in my arms. "Little does she know what? That you took one look at me and went screaming in the other direction?" Lynne bats her long eyelashes at me.

I swat her on her ass in retaliation. "Not hardly." Then I lean down and kiss her.

For long moments, we do nothing more than inhale each other while we sway together to the music that's pulsating in the air between her heartbeat and mine. When I let Lynne up for a breath, her smile is so wide her dimple makes an appearance. "That's right. You had to be lured onto the dance floor. Hmm, makes a girl wonder."

"Wonder what?" But I'm stunned as Lynne's luscious body begins to shift and move. "God, you dance and there's such beauty. I could watch it forever." The words slip from me unbidden.

She spins around, her energy high. "Then come with me."

I step closer. "Here?"

She shakes her head. "No. To Nantucket." She bites her lower lip anxiously.

"You're serious?"

"I never thought to ask someone. I never cared enough to look for an escort. But you? You're perfect." Lynne goes on to say something else, but I'm frozen.

I react without thinking of anything but myself. "The answer's no," I tell her bluntly.

The look on her face is like tearing the wings off a butterfly. It's littered with humiliation. "Of course. I'm so sorry for asking. You know, I just remembered something I have to do before tomorrow. I should probably go." Lynne races to head back into the elevator.

I should let her go, but I can't. All I can remember is the expression on her face when she shared her agony with me this morning. Just as she's about to reach the elevator, I call out, "It's because of work, *mon étoile*. I cannot get away with that kind of notice." It's a lie, the first damn one I'll tell her. But to keep this kind of secret from her, I'll lie every single day. I'll lie to her face if I have to.

It's the only way I'll have enough time to store up memories before she'll eventually tire of it and find someone more worthy to love.

Back still to me, she murmurs, "Of course it is. Still, I should go."

I approach, hiding behind a demeanor I use every night of my life —one where everything is focused on everything but me. "Stay," I coax. My hand passes over her hair. I pray she doesn't notice how it trembles.

She wavers. "If you're certain?"

I nod decisively. "I am. Besides, we bought groceries. What am I going to do with all this food unless you stay to have dinner with me?"

Without another word, Lynne goes to work to prepare our meal. While she does, I grab a bottle of wine and turn on some music to eliminate the silence that's wedged its way between us.

~

I PRESS HER LEGS APART, ruthlessly holding her wide as I swipe my tongue through her dampness. I refuse to let her touch me tonight, despite her pleas.

Lynne is stretched out on my bed like a sacrifice. Her hands are gripping the sheets like she'd like to be touching me, but I forced her hands to the side a while ago with a whispered "No touching."

Not tonight. Not after what she said. I think I might break otherwise.

"You taste divine," I murmur the accolade. Turning my head to the side, I brush kisses up the inside of her thigh.

Lynne's eyes pop open when I shift back to get a condom to slide on. "Don't stop." There's a desperation in her voice that catches me low in the gut.

"I wasn't planning on stopping." I hold up two fingers. In the shadows, the square packet to protect us both gleams.

"Oh." I can feel her embarrassment pulsate off her body in waves of heat.

Stretching out on top of her, I frame her face in my hands before trailing kisses from her cheek to her ear. "Lynne, what is it?"

Her head turns away, "I—you—" But her lips clamp together.

I trail my fingers all over her body, but when she gathers her emotions, her whispered words cause me to freeze. "You said you'd never lie to me, but you are. I don't know what I did. I just asked you to come to a wedding with me as my date. All you had to do was say no." The moonlight causes the tears on her face to glisten as she rolls to her side.

Away from me.

Agonizing pain sears through me. "*Non, mon étoile.* That's not what I was..." I reach out to touch her shoulder, but she's as stiff as a board.

"Maybe I should just leave since I'm going in the morning anyway." Lynne sits up with her back to me. Panic assails me. As sure as I know my name, I know if she walks out the door, a part of me will go with her—possibly the last part that hasn't been damaged by the past. I've spent close to half my life recovering from a few years of mistakes. But the mingled feelings of shame and guilt still rear their ugly head.

And tonight, I took them out on a woman who had nothing to do with any of it. Her loyalty, vulnerability, and openheartedness are what attracted me to her in the first place, and now, I'm punishing her for what? A wrong word choice?

I should be shot.

"Don't go," I rasp out. Crawling across the bed, I place my hand on her wrist. "Please."

"Will you tell me why?" Her voice is clear and strong.

Knowing I'm going to have to tell her to keep her terrifies me. But I know I can't dodge this bullet. "Not now." In time. Perhaps. Hopefully never.

Her breathing evens out. "Fine. Let's get some sleep." Lynne lies down, curling into herself.

And as I lie behind her, I know it's wrong. We should be twined together. Amazing how twenty-four hours earlier, I was terrified of spending the night holding her, but I know what holding her feels like.

It's the answer to dreams I don't deserve.

Cautiously, I slide my hand over her hip and pull myself toward her. Curling my knees beneath the back of hers, I try to surround her with my body heat, the very thing I kept from her when I tried to touch her earlier.

Eventually, Lynne relaxes enough to ease back against me, and my breath accelerates like I just stepped off the dance floor downstairs.

How appropriate.

25

MARCO

Once her breathing evens out, and I'm certain she's asleep, I bury my head against the back of her neck where her soft hair ends. And ashamed, I tell her the truth because I promised her no lies.

"*Maman*—our mother—was very beautiful. When she died, the world went dark. For a while, we were too wrapped in our grief to think beyond that. But like you said earlier, with time pain eases. And there I was with nothing but a cottage and a little brother to support.

"I drove to Paris to answer an ad for modeling, never believing I would be selected, but I was. I could not believe my fortune. I thought I was too old, but they assured me I was perfect.

"I was to show up and precisely *six heures du soir* at this *grande* estate. I was given an outfit to wear—a tuxedo. *Mon Dieu*, to this day, I cannot bear to wear them." I swallow hard, smell the perfection of Lynne's scent before going on.

"It wasn't a modeling job, but an audition of sorts. And I'm so... ashamed to say I took it."

Lynne shifts a bit but settles. I wait a few moments before whispering my ultimate shame. "Simon had dreams, Lynne. And it became my responsibility to be able to provide him the ability to seek them. But once it started, I knew I'd need enough money to start over. After all, how do you explain a five-year gap in employment?" I sigh, my breath ruffling the back of her thick hair. "It's shameful, and I can't look you in the eyes and tell you this because a woman who has the universe as her path will always think there was another way, some other way. But I was desperate. And alone. So, so, alone."

Kissing the back of her head, tears trickle down my face that are absorbed by her thick hair. "Even when she kissed me after she was through with me, before I was sent back to my quarters until the next time I was summoned, I was alone. All I had was the knowledge I was using the one asset I had—my body—to buy Simon's future. And maybe, my own chance at redemption."

I brush a kiss on her shoulder, light as air so as not to wake her during my confession. "So, you see, *mon étoile*, when you asked me to escort you to the wedding, that was why I reacted poorly. It wasn't you I was rejecting; it was my past. I don't want anything to ever tarnish you—" My heart pounds so hard it's a wonder she can't hear it. "—*parce que j'étais un escorte*. A body for hire. It's how I had enough money to come seek a new life in America, how I bought the building. Why I won't ever touch the money Bristol invests for us. But it's why I will let you take that small bit and try to make it grow so I can give it away—to do good with it much like you did with your job at Lockwood, like you do with your own money. But I trust you to do your best. Me though. I am not worthy of it. Of you."

My voice is shredded by the time I'm done. Pulling Lynne close, my heart aches knowing what I want is to make love to her one more time before she has to leave in the morning, but I know she needs her rest after the emotional turmoil I've put her through in the last few days. She's already given up days to be with me and will be insanely busy from the moment she touches down on the island.

My lips touch her cheek before my eyes finally flutter shut, exhausted.

My heart misses her already and she's not even gone.

THE NEXT MORNING, I wake as she's getting dressed. Wearing only a pair of red silky tap pants and a matching demi-cup bra, Lynne drops her arms to her sides, and I make a growling noise from the bed.

She spins around, startled. Her eyes are red-rimmed. Just as she's about to speak, I throw back the covers. "What is wrong?" I demand.

Her lips curve in contrast to the tears dripping from her eyes. "I'm going to miss you, and I'm not sure how to handle that."

I narrow my eyes as I make my approach. But her azure eyes are meeting mine directly. "You're serious?" I ask incredulously.

She nods, before reaching for the flowing knee-length circle skirt she wore yesterday. Slipping it on and then pulling a red T-shirt over her head, she steps into a pair of matching flats before shoving various items into her oversized purse. A quick glance at her watch makes her gasp. "The car will be here soon."

I snag the pants I shucked off the night before and slide them on to lead her safely downstairs. "I'm going to miss you," I tell her honestly.

She hesitates before reiterating, "The offer's still open."

We enter the elevator, and I press the Down button. Rather than use these last few moments on words, I pull her into my arms and kiss her. I need this contact to last me until I can hold her again, until I can solidify what it is between us.

The elevator stops with its usual jarring bang. Lynne breaks our kiss. "I still find it rather rude the way it interrupts us."

"This morning, I could not agree with you more." We step outside, and her car is waiting. "Will you text me to let me know you've landed safely, *mon étoile*?"

"Yes." Brushing a kiss against my lips, she then kisses my forehead and leans down to kiss my chest over my heart. "Maybe that will help remind you," she says mysteriously.

Of what? I wonder, but I don't get the chance to ask. The driver is leaping out to assist Lynne into the car. The door closes, but within seconds, she rolls the window down.

"Let me know if you change your mind. It's just a casual beach wedding: shirt, slacks, no shoes."

"Perhaps." I'm perplexed about why she's reminding me again about the attire when it's doubtful I'll change my mind.

"Marco?" Lynne stretches her hand out the window.

I immediately reach for her wrist and lift it to my lips. I need the whiff of her scent to last me. "Yes?"

"I left something for you on your phone." Pulling her hand back, she instructs the driver, "Let's go."

Wondering what it is, I step back and wave once as the car pulls out of the gate. Finally, I go back inside and take the interminable elevator ride back up. Once I enter the main living space, I spy my cell phone on the kitchen counter. Unable to wait, I find an unread text message from Lynne, and I open it.

Then I grab the counter for support as my legs give out from under me.

Tapping the screen is a selfie of us in bed just a few hours earlier. Lynne is kissing my head, which is resting on her chest. And captioned beneath it she wrote, *I told you once, we can't regret everything and everyone that led us here. If I did, then I wouldn't have the strength and patience to be the woman who fits in your arms. And that is worse than anything that ever happened. It won't be easy, but I love your idea. We'll talk more when I return. And remember, the only person you have to forgive is yourself. In life, that's all we should expect from one another; don't you think? XOXO*

Stumbling to the sofa, I feel violently ill and somehow so elated I can fly at the same time.

She knows and she's not running.

After a long while of absorbing this, I curse myself for letting her leave. Shoving to my feet, I text Louie to determine our schedule the next few days and if I can get away.

Then, I storm into the bedroom and stop short at the foot of the bed. Closing my eyes, I whisper a prayer of thanks, something I haven't done since I was a young man. It's been so long, I could have sworn I forgot how. I should have known it would come back to me as easily as the moves of a dance.

As I stand there, I feel humbled as parts of my soul hidden in the dark for so long are exposed to light for the first time.

And I feel free.

26

LYNNE

Fortunately, I had everything packed before I went to Marco's last night, so I just raced home and changed. Ryan called my cell phone from the limo about five minutes after I managed to drag everything to the lobby.

After the driver loads everything into the trunk, I throw myself into the back where Ryan and Jared are sipping mimosas. Ryan takes one look at me and mutters, "Uh-oh. I know that look. Jared, pour her a drink."

"Jared, if you add cranberry, I might try to steal you away from your husband," I try to joke, but tears prick my eyes.

Jared quickly mixes the cocktail before sliding across the seat with it. Handing me my drink, he reaches for his own before wrapping an arm around my shoulders. "Is this more than your best friend is getting married tears?"

"So much more." I lift the drink away from my body as the driver takes a tight turn. "Cheers, gentlemen. I finally met a man."

Ryan's savage "I'll kill him for hurting you" makes me kick out my well-shod foot.

"He didn't hurt me—not in the way you mean at least." I take a long drink to fortify myself. "He just makes me feel so much, I can't keep it all inside." While that's completely true, what Marco shared was for my heart to bear and isn't up for public consumption.

Ryan relaxes a bit. "You should have invited him to the wedding. Then I could have checked him out."

I roll my eyes. "Please. Save the investigation work for your brother. Caleb's so much better at it."

"Where do you think I get all my information?" Ryan drawls. He points at Jared. "Where do you think he gets all of his?" Jared is a partner in one of Manhattan's most lucrative law firms.

"You are not looking into his background," I declare firmly.

"We'll see," Ryan says smugly.

I debate between tossing the rest of my drink in his face and finishing it. But I know the way gossip spreads in this family he'll know by dinner who I mean, so I tip my head back and sip.

"I'm glad you're flying up with us anyway," Ryan says seriously.

"Why? Going to give me advice on my love life the entire flight?" I say scathingly.

"No. That's just an added bonus." Tugging my hand, Ryan pulls me away from Jared and across the seat into his own strong arms. "I missed you so much, Lynne. The office isn't the same without you."

I burst into tears.

"Oh crap. Jared, do something," Ry says frantically.

"What am I supposed to do? You're the one who started this," Jared lectures his husband.

I start giggling uncontrollably.

"Oh, you're falling for certain. It's a clear case of PMS to me."

"Post-Marco Syndrome. Sounds about right," I mutter to myself.

Or so I think.

"Marco? As in Marco Houde? Bristol's brother-in-law?" Ryan says carefully. His arms haven't relaxed. If anything, they've tightened even more around me.

"As in Corinna's ex?" Jared adds even more cautiously.

"As in Corinna, Colby, and everyone in the family's *friend*," I stress. "That I met the other night when we went to Jenna's bachelorette party."

"Isn't he like fifteen years older than you?" Ryan shouts.

"Less than that." It's the truth. It's closer to thirteen and a half years.

"Not by much," he shoots back.

"I'm sorry. What's the age difference between Jenna and Finn?"

"That girl's putting ideas in your head," Ryan grouses.

"Damn hot ones. You've met Finn," I remind him.

"She's got you there, Ry," Jared laughs.

A particularly nasty jolt on the highway has me and Ryan skidding across the seat. "Ugh," I grunt.

"That's just how I feel about you and Marco."

I swat him. "How well do you know him?" I demand.

"Not well," he concedes. "But you're you, Lynne. There's no one on the planet who's going to be good enough for you. Even if Caleb was still unmarried, I wouldn't think *he* was good enough for you."

I open my mouth and close it several times before I'm able to push out, "Damn you, Ryan." Hot tears flood my eyes before spilling down my face again.

"It was the right business move, but I miss you every day. Expect to have me glued to your side when Jenna's not with you. And if Marco does shows up, well, he should expect to be put through the wringer."

A laugh bubbles up despite the tears as we pull into the airport departures. "Why do I suspect that's why he's not coming?"

Jared chortles as he exits the car, Ryan right behind him. I take a deep breath and follow them to sort out bags that are heading to Caleb's private jet which is smaller than Ryan's and can land on Nantucket.

The three of us quickly pass through Security and board the plane. After takeoff, we all become engrossed in our own computers. I check the schedule I created one more time. Just a few more hours and I won't have a lot of time to think about Marco, I think desperately.

Because I'm terrified.

It's been hours since I left his place, and I haven't heard anything. Not a single word.

Did I ruin our fragile beginning by admitting I'd heard what he whispered to me?

I let out an involuntary "Umph" as Ryan accidentally kicks me when he sits down across from me. Glaring at him, I close my laptop lid. "You rang?"

"Work time is over," he singsongs.

"For your information, I was checking the schedule I created for the next few days," I inform him haughtily.

Ryan groans, drawing a smile from me. "My love, come save me. Lynne created a schedule for the beach."

Jared joins us. "Lynne, ignore him. He's behaving like a two-year-old."

"And that's different from a normal workday for him, how?" I jibe, getting some of my own back.

Ryan holds his hands to his chest, as if he suffered a mortal blow. "I'm wounded. Now, tell me how you've organized our lives..."

I shoot him a quelling glance.

"He means how you carefully organized the events so we have time for all of the fun," Jared interprets.

"Like use the restroom," Ryan whimpers.

Carefully avoiding Jared's legs, I kick Ryan soundly.

"Damn. You had to wear pointed-toe shoes." He rubs his shin.

"I've flown with you before. I know how to provide myself with amusement." I glance at my nails, glad we're getting them done tomorrow. "It's a free-for-all."

"Just think." Ryan bats his deep brown eyes at me. "This could be you one day."

I shake my head furiously. "No, this will never be me."

"Why not?" Ryan demands, suddenly serious. "Don't you want to get married?"

"Maybe. But I don't want this kind of pomp and circumstance."

"What would you want?"

"You want me to plan a wedding out of thin air?"

Ryan laughs. "Haven't we all done that?" Before I can lambast him, he reminds me, "Cass says we do."

"True." I think about it for a few moments. "I think I'd want something small with family and friends. I want it to be about the vows we're about to take, not the outrageousness of the ceremony."

"In other words, you want it to be the complete opposite of ours," Jared says dryly.

I flush hotly. "I didn't mean..."

He holds up a hand. "We had our reasons for our wedding being that way, Lynne. And it was beautiful because all of those people got to witness me tying my life to Ryan's. But you're right. When you get married—"

"If," I correct.

"When," he argues, his lawyer side emerging. "Each ceremony should be unique to the couple. When it's your time, it will be."

I open my mouth to say more, but before I can, the pilot is announcing our approach. We all buckle in before moments later, we're touching down.

Outside of the window, a large SUV is waiting for us on the edge of the runway. Both the driver and passenger get out, and I spy wild blonde curls dancing in the breeze.

I want off this plane. Now.

I fly down the stairs once they're lowered and haul across the tarmac into Em's arms. They close around me tightly as Caleb walks past us to greet his brother and brother-in-law. She's still holding me even after the guys have loaded our luggage. "Will you tell me?" Em finally whispers.

I think long and hard before I shake my head no against her shoulder. I do pull back far enough to tell her something she'll understand better than anyone else because she helped raise me and Jenna, and she changed her life for the better. "He doesn't think he's worth it."

A lifetime of memories swirl in her eyes before she simply tugs me forward into her arms again without words needing to be spoken.

27

LYNNE

"I recognize the expression on your face." Em comes up next to me as I lean against the rail of the guest apartment the day of the wedding. "In fact, I drew several pictures of myself in this very spot with it."

I open my mouth and try to deny it. "After four days?"

She wraps an arm around my waist. "It took Phil and Jason an instant. Ali and Keene a night. Connections are made when they're made, darling girl. It doesn't mean you rush into anything but don't deny the feelings."

I rest my head on hers as the ocean air soothes me. "What if it's one-sided, Em? What if he doesn't feel the same way?" Giving voice to my biggest fear leaches some of the poison from it somehow.

She turns me to face her. "We've stood here together too many times to count since the first time we met, and despite the fact I hate the reason why, I'm honored you've become another daughter for me to love, Lynne."

Tears sting my eyes. "Me too."

"I'll remind you of the same thing I told you about the boy in college and then the one in grad school." Her hand pushes a few stands of hair away from my face. "Take your time. Know your heart.

Love freely. And if it doesn't work out, come home. We always love you for who you are."

"I know. But this time it's different." I pull away and lean against the railing again.

"Why?"

"Because Marco's part of this family in his own right."

Corinna's voice comes from behind us, making me jump. "And knowing you're worried about that, about him, already assures me this is going to be fine. Em, can I have a moment with Lynne?"

"Of course." Em squeezes my shoulder and slips back inside to help Jenna get ready. In the distance, music can be heard from the main house while vendors are setting up the arbor on the beach under Phil's guidance.

It's a beautiful day for a wedding. And soon, I'll slide out of this mood and into a festive one.

I haven't heard from Marco since I sent the text. I thought it would be easier for him to know I heard his confession, but obviously I was wrong. So, so wrong.

I declare, "I'm not sure how much I'll be around after the wedding."

"What do you mean? You just got home." Corinna's concerned.

Home. What an incredible word. Yes, I've made my home with the family here, but what about what Marco needs? What about his need for security, for acceptance? Unable to express my thought, I focus on the crashing waves.

Corinna's hand smooths up and down my back. "In just a few short days, you managed to get closer to Marco than anyone."

I let out a choked laugh. "I don't think he thanks me for it. It's probably better for him if I go back to what I do best—being a part of this family from a distance."

Corinna opens her mouth to argue, but the words that come out aren't hers. "I thought you were happy to be home the night we ate with your Suzie-Q, *mon étoile*. Was I wrong?"

My body locks. I'm unable to make myself turn around to face Marco. *He's here*, my heart whispers. All I can absorb is Corinna moving away toward him. She says something softly, words swallowed by the waves. But his "I promise" rings out.

What? What is he promising? Not to cause a scene at Jenna's wedding? Of course, my logical mind reminds me, he could have avoided that simply by not showing up.

"Whenever I think of a family wedding, I remember Simon's wedding to Bristol. There were four of us." Marco steps up next to me. When he does, the scents of the beach fade as I greedily inhale the scent of his cologne and his skin. "This would be considered by some to be a circus."

I turn my head to the side and immediately regret it. Dressed in an ocean-blue silk shirt and black slacks, Marco's perfectly dressed for the wedding—especially if he plans on escorting the maid of honor. Facing forward, I can't prevent the curve of my lips as Phil takes off down the beach after a long piece of wayward tulle. "When is a Freeman event not a circus?"

"An excellent question. But not an answer to my earlier question." Marco reaches over and lays his hand on mine. "Do you really want to travel again, *mon étoile*?"

Staring into the horizon, I blame the blistering sun for causing the hot tears that begin to trickle across my cheeks. "No. But it's better if I go." Now would be preferable, but I can't do that to Jenna.

Marco tugs me until I'm facing him. "Why?"

A simple question with a million answers. "Because." *Think, Lynne.* "I...need to support Bristol." *I need to leave you to with people who care for you.* My eyes dart back to the crashing waves.

"Do you think you could give it a few weeks?"

A few weeks. My head drops as I imagine what that would mean. If I hadn't already started the first steps of love with this man, I would welcome the weeks he's offering. But now? "I don't know," I hedge. Many more nights like my last with Marco and I might be a shell by the time our affair ends.

Then how do I survive?

He leans down and presses his lips against each cheek. *Here comes his goodbye.* I brace myself mentally. "It may take weeks to find someone to work the floor of the club so I can travel with you, Lynne. I can come back and check on it when you have to travel to France."

I'm a statue in his arms while he struggles for words. "I'm not strong enough to face those ghosts yet. Over time, perhaps. After all —" He pulls back to admire me in my short silk robe. "—you come to this place you abhor to celebrate love. How strong you are to do that, *mon étoile*."

"Hold on." I lift my hand, and Marco immediately captures it. Lifting it, he presses his lips to the inside of my wrist. "You haven't said a word to me in days. And now you're here. Why?"

"I met you in the place I built to hide in the dark, and with one smile, you lit up the entire room. I already thought you were beautiful before I held your body against mine while we danced."

Marco yanks me toward him. "But nothing holds a candle to the gift you gave me when you left me that morning. Acceptance for who I am, for who I was."

"Yes." My voice is ragged.

"Then if you plan on traveling the world again, I accept this. I accept you, Lynne Bradbury, however you can give yourself. I just want to experience the light with you." Leaning down, his breath sends shivers along my spine when he whispers, "There are many places in this world where we can hold each other and dance."

"And if I stay? What happens then?"

For long moments, we stand so still I think it's all over. Then Marco picks up my hand. Laying it over his heart, I feel the deep beat. He begins swaying our bodies gently back and forth.

I'm scared to speak, scared to let go, when all I want is my head to be free to explore what my heart is scared it already knows.

This man is everything.

"We will dance no matter where we are, *mon étoile*. The music will come from here." Marco lays a hand on first his heart before moving it over to mine. "It matters not where we stand. All that is important to me is us. Together. Trying. *N'est-ce pas?*" His face is vulnerable.

Sliding my hand to the back of his neck, I whisper, "*Oui.*"

His breath shudders out as he enfolds me next in his arms. Naturally, we begin to sway together as he confesses, "I could not reach out until I spoke with my family. I needed to share with them what I told you."

I pull back so I can brush the dampness from the shadows beneath Marco's eyes. "And when you're ready, you can share what happened. For now, you only have one thing to worry about."

Even as his face starts to relax, an arrogant brow rises. "What's that?"

"I may be called upon to sing. I tried to warn you, it's going to be terrible." Rising up on the balls of my feet, I brush my lips across his. "You may feel differently about me after."

"Lynne, I cannot imagine my feelings differing simply because you bleat like *un mouton*."

A sheep. I whack him in the shoulder before he captures my face in his hands. "You have freed my heart. For now, we live in our present." What he leaves unsaid, and what I don't need to hear because his lips on mine speak for me, is that when the time is right, we will determine a future.

Together.

Someday.

And no one will have the right to judge us in the world we create together because the only people who matter in it are me and Marco.

EPILOGUE
MARCO - ONE YEAR LATER

In a day, your whole life can change. From one night to the next, I was alone in a sea of people. I believed myself crippled by my past to realizing I cradle love closer to my heart because of it. In a week, love's foundation was built. In a month, it was impossible for me to deny.

As days passed, as the sun rose and set on New York, as we came and went traveling around the globe, nothing was more precious than the first time I held Lynne in my arms and whispered, "I love you." My soul felt reborn when she wrapped her arms around me and whispered, "I love you too. But looking back, I think I knew that the first time you lied to me and then explained why. How could I not love you?"

In a year's worth of days, we've argued as much as we've loved, but more than that, we've held each other while we did nothing but sway to the music life's created all around us.

I'm a lucky bastard, and I know it.

"Are you certain everything is in place?" I confirm with Louie as I fiddle with my bow tie before I let the ends hang helplessly.

"Man, everything is perfect. Exactly the way you planned," he grumbles.

"We planned," I correct him. "I want everything exactly how Lynne wants it."

Simon's laughter rings out as he chases Alex around my living room. "I'll fix that bow tie again once I get Alex's done."

"Great. It's my wedding and I have to wait for the ring bearer to get dressed," I joke.

"At least he didn't have an accident on your rug," Simon reminds me.

"I take it back. Fix your son."

"Worse comes to worst, Marco will just start a new trend." Louie's smile is sly.

"What's that?" Simon snags Alex. "Got you, you rascal!"

Alex giggles.

"Undressing for his bride before the ceremony." While Louie and Simon laugh, I pretend to give great thought to this idea. But no, there's symbolism to wearing a tuxedo for my fiancée, my Lynne, the woman my world orbits around. "I want everything to be perfect."

We all pause as we hear the clicking of heels and the swooshing of a dress. "As long as you meet her at the end of the aisle, everything will be," Corinna reassures me. She tips her head back to receive Colby's kiss before she approaches. "Now, stop fidgeting and let me fix that bow tie. As one of your groomsmen, it's the least I can do."

I stand perfectly still while Corinna's fingers make quick work of the silk, flipping and twisting it until it lies perfectly around my neck. "Did I ever say thank you, *ma chère amie*?" I murmur softly.

Her warm eyes lift to mine. "For what?"

"For being generous with your heart in a time when you didn't have to be. Then later, for doing it again with someone who didn't expect it." I lean down and brush a kiss across her cheek softly. "We both appreciate your friendship very much, Cori."

"Of course."

"You know you will always have a place in my heart."

Shakily, Corinna presses a hand against my chest. "And you in mine. *Toujours.*" Always.

"That's how long I'll love her," I whisper.

"Then you finally found what I wanted you to have. What I found all those years ago." She steps back and grins wickedly. "Now, Colby, where's Lynne's gift for Marco?"

He steps forward and holds out a small black bag. "I'm sorry, man, but there was a lot of cackling going on," Colby apologizes.

"'In case of emergency.' What does she think is going to happen?" Reaching inside, I pull out a handful of silk. And roar with laughter. "That minx. I should have sent her a vibr—"

Simon coughs and points at his son.

"Vibrant bouquet."

"Nice save," Monty declares as he walks off the elevator with Evangeline in tow.

Evangeline takes one look at what I'm holding and trips on her heels. "Oh. I knew I loved Lynne. But this? Brilliant."

Corinna brushes her fingers on her dress before blowing on them. "We taught her well."

"I actually came up to steal Alex, but if you're opening gifts, it can wait." Evangeline hooks an arm around Monty's waist.

I slide my hand back into the bag and pull out a custom jewelry box and a card. Placing the box aside, I slip out the card. On the cover is a couple dancing beneath the night sky.

Inside, all it says is "I wonder if dancing as a Mrs. will be any different? Let's dance and find out. I love you. - L"

I tuck the card beneath my arm while I pick up the box. Opening it, I find a pair of star-shaped cufflinks made of rubies whose color match the fall of the velvet downstairs in Redemption. "Will someone help me?" I ask the room at large, not wanting to let go of the card until I have to.

Quickly switching out cufflinks, I smooth my jacket down. Placing the card in front of so many others we've received, I announce to my closest family and friends, "It's time, *n'est-ce pas?*"

I hug Louie and my brother and fist-bump Alex. I shake Colby's hand, offer an arm to Corinna, kiss Evangeline, slap Monty's shoulder, and gesture everyone to the elevator.

I'm beyond ready.

~

Bristol walks down the aisle first, her dress a light rose. Next comes Emily, in a deeper shade. Finally, Jenna, pregnant with her first child. She reaches out and squeezes her Finn's hand as she passes by him. Their love is evident, even to the most casual of observers.

Then everyone stands. And my breath catches.

Lynne showed me the first dress Em made for her when she was sixteen—an original Emily Freeman design that was a gift. Today, she wears another, still simplistic in its beauty, highlighting her curves. But today, it's dusted in crystals that look like stars.

As Ryan escorts her down the aisle, I catch sight of the ruby resting temporarily on Lynne's right hand. Oh, how surprised she was when she opened her door in Paris and found me there, I remember fondly. Instead of focusing on being in the city that almost destroyed me, I focused on the woman who saved me—her shocked face before dropping to one knee after she opened the door. Before I could get a word out, Lynne whispered, "Whatever the question is, my answer is yes."

Swooping her up in my arms, I kicked the door shut behind me. I did manage to ask her properly after making love to her with my ring warming her finger in her suite at the Ritz.

That trip, we put my ghosts to rest as well as made new memories to be able to pull out again someday. But not now. Not when Ryan is holding out Lynne's hand to mine. When I touch her fingers, all the excitement, the passion, and the certainty from our first meeting coalesce.

"*Mon étoile,* you look exquisite," I murmur as we approach both the judge who will perform the legal part of our ceremony and Charlie Henderson, an avuncular family friend who will conduct the celebratory portion.

"As do you." Her bright blue eyes are shining with so much love, I know I'll never feel hollow again.

I slip my arm around her waist and tug her in front of me. Almost naturally, she begins to sway in my embrace when my hand finds her stomach.

Whispering softly, I tell Lynne, "I love you."

She looks over her shoulder. For just a moment, I'm transported to that first night where we danced together on this very spot. Her "I love you" makes me appreciate every step of my life was choreographed to lead me to this moment.

And as Charlie asks the intimate gathering of family and friends around us if anyone objects to our marriage, I'm curious if the child we found out we were having last week will grow up loving to dance.

I certainly hope so.

~

The End

THE END

WHERE TO GET HELP

When I first wrote Corinna Freeman's story in Free to Breathe and introduced the character of Marco Houde, the darkness of his dark past flooded me. After all, it isn't unusual for two lost souls to connect for a brief time, if only to help each other along the path to their healing.

There are many people in this world that believe the choices Marco made are their only options due to financial, emotional, or physically threatening situations. Some elect to try prostitution because they feel there is now a greater acceptance and legal protection due to decriminalization in some regions of the world.

Prostitution is considered by many to be a human rights violation. There are an estimated 40 million people in prostitution worldwide. The overwhelming majority are women and girls. Organizations like SPACE (Survivors of Prostitution Abuse Calling for Enlightenment) give voice to women who have survived the harsh reality of prostitution. When I read the testimonials on this site and many others before diving into Marco's story, my heart crumbled at the tenacity and strength people have not simply to endure but to thrive. But the most important thing I learned was, if you need assistance, reach out to someone you trust.

I write romance because I believe everyone deserves to find their life partner, someone who can appreciate them and not be judgmental of the choices they made. I'm just thrilled for a man who has lived most of his life in the shadows, done things he regrets, he found it in the light of a star.

ACKNOWLEDGMENTS

To my beloved husband. For always loving me even when there were days when I felt unlovable. And for championing what I do.

To my son, I've said this a million times; all that matters is trying. I'll love you no matter what.

To my mother and father, you raised me to be a determined fighter regardless of the circumstances. I love you both.

Jen, I can't wait to hug you in person! It's been thirty years this year since we became friends. I realize the symbolism of us climbing that mountain every time I think about it. We were, and are, unstoppable.

To my Meows. Forever my inspiration, irreplaceable in my heart. Your love and friendship mean everything to me. I miss all of you each and every day.

Ah, Sandra Depukat from One Love Editing. You always push me exactly where I need to be. XOXO Also, I need to thank "J" profusely for refreshing my gutter French. Give him a big smooch for me.

To Holly Malgieri, from Holly's Red Hot Reviews, a.k.a. my twin, I could hear your "YESSSS!" the moment this landed in your inbox. Love you!

To Amy Queau, from QDesigns, from the first Amaryllis cover to now, thank you for picking the nuances out of my brain even when I can't quite verbalize it.

To Gel, at Tempting Illustrations, thank you, thank you, thank you!

To the fantastic team at Foreword PR, thank you for everything you've ever done since the first Amaryllis book was published!

Linda Russell, have I hurt your brain yet? Love you forever!

To my Musketeers. You know who you are. #nowandforever

To Amy Rhodes and Dawn Hurst, you are just that amazing!

Sue Henn, you're not getting off so easily. I'm so grateful you sent that message. Remember, just dance.

And to everyone who has joined me on the Amaryllis journey, I love you! It has been amazing stepping back into the Amaryllis Series. I thought it appropriate I answer this question once and for all...

Yes. There will be more stories from the Amaryllis Universe. I will bring back the original characters as I tell stories of others. But trust me, you will still see updates from our friends and the town of Collyer, Connecticut.

ABOUT THE AUTHOR

Tracey Jerald knew she was meant to be a writer when she would re-write the ending of books in her head when she was a young girl growing up in southern Connecticut. It wasn't long before she was typing alternate endings and extended epilogues "just for fun".

After college in Florida, where she obtained a degree in Criminal Justice, Tracey traded the world of law and order for IT. Her work for a world-wide internet startup transferred her to Northern Virginia where she met her husband in what many call their own happily ever after. They have one son.

When she's not busy with her family or writing, Tracey can be found in her home in north Florida drinking coffee, reading, training for a runDisney event, or feeding her addiction to HGTV.

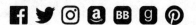